NEUROSCIENCE RESEARCH PROGRESS

A NEW APPROACH TO ETIOPATHOGENESIS OF DEPRESSION

NEUROPLASTICITY

NEUROSCIENCE RESEARCH PROGRESS

Additional books in this series can be found on Nova's website
under the Series tab.

Additional E-books in this series can be found on Nova's website
under the E-books tab.

NEUROSCIENCE RESEARCH PROGRESS

A NEW APPROACH TO ETIOPATHOGENESIS OF DEPRESSION

NEUROPLASTICITY

I. TAYFUN UZBAY

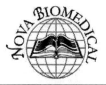

Nova Science Publishers, Inc.
New York

For permission to use material from this book please contact us:
Telephone 631-231-7269; Fax 631-231-8175
Web Site: http://www.novapublishers.com

NOTICE TO THE READER

The Publisher has taken reasonable care in the preparation of this book, but makes no expressed or implied warranty of any kind and assumes no responsibility for any errors or omissions. No liability is assumed for incidental or consequential damages in connection with or arising out of information contained in this book. The Publisher shall not be liable for any special, consequential, or exemplary damages resulting, in whole or in part, from the readers' use of, or reliance upon, this material. Any parts of this book based on government reports are so indicated and copyright is claimed for those parts to the extent applicable to compilations of such works.

Independent verification should be sought for any data, advice or recommendations contained in this book. In addition, no responsibility is assumed by the publisher for any injury and/or damage to persons or property arising from any methods, products, instructions, ideas or otherwise contained in this publication.

This publication is designed to provide accurate and authoritative information with regard to the subject matter covered herein. It is sold with the clear understanding that the Publisher is not engaged in rendering legal or any other professional services. If legal or any other expert assistance is required, the services of a competent person should be sought. FROM A DECLARATION OF PARTICIPANTS JOINTLY ADOPTED BY A COMMITTEE OF THE AMERICAN BAR ASSOCIATION AND A COMMITTEE OF PUBLISHERS.

Additional color graphics may be available in the e-book version of this book.

Library of Congress Cataloging-in-Publication Data

Uzbay, Tayfun.
  A new approach to etiopathogenesis of depression : neuroplasticity /
Tayfun Uzbay.
      p. cm.
  Includes bibliographical references and index.
  ISBN 978-1-61209-554-7 (softcover : alk. paper)
  1. Neuroplasticity. 2. Depression, Mental--Etiology. 3. Depression,
Mental--Diagnosis. I. Title.
  QP363.3.U93 2011
  616.85'27--dc22
                        2011006700

Published by Nova Science Publishers, Inc.†New York

Contents

Preface

Our knowledge about brain functions is still limited in the era of knowledge and communication. Consequently rational drug treatment for diseases that are directly related with brain functions like Alzheimer's disease, schizophrenia, Parkinson's disease, substance dependence has not been possible yet. Recently more resources are allocated in technologically and scientifically developed countries to the treatment of brain related diseases. Many scientists also state that this period will be dominated by scientific brain research.

Depression is a mood disorder that may appear in any part of life and its prevalence is increasing. Impairment of life quality at the level that causes loss of workforce and suicidal outcome in some cases increases its importance. Monoamine hypothesis that was proposed to be related with the cause of depression is still valid today although there are problems to be solved regarding definitive diagnosis of depression and rational pharmacotherapy. This forces the scientists to form alternative and more valid hypothesis about the etiology of depression.

Neuroplasticity can be defined shortly as the adaptability of neuron to internal and external stimuli. It was believed formerly that neurons can not regenerate. Recent studies on central nervous system have clearly found that neurons have the property to regenerate and repair themselves as other cells do. This observation makes the major contribution to the emergence of neuroplasticity hypothesis as well as it is a critical point for the diagnosis and treatment of diseases related with central nervous system.

In recent years, contribution of especially stress induced neuroplastic changes in brain to depression besides other diseases with central origin is indicated. Intensity and importance of research on this topic is increasing. Neuroplasticity hypothesis of depression has the potential to make important contributions to the diagnosis of depression as well as it may be helpful in the explanation of the drug effects can not be explained by neurochemical mechanisms. Also, it seems that it may lead to the development of new and more effective drugs for depression and entrance of this drug to treatment in a short time.

In this book we tried to acquaint readers about the neuroplasticity hypothesis especially in the context of depression. Knowledge covered in this book is as much as the literature reviewed about this topic. Neuroplasticity is a dynamic topic. It is possible that additional concepts emerge in parallel to new developments and this subject is reshaped.

Dr. Hakan Kayir has made valuable contributions during the writing process of this book. I thank to Dr. Kayir for his eager efforts during composition and publication of this book.

Chapter 1

General Concepts and Information about Central Nervous System

Neuron and Its Structure

Neruon is the functional and structural unit of the nervous system. It is a specialized cell that receives, transmits and emits neuronal stimuli. It has special features in regards to both structure and functions, different from other cell types. Neuron, as shown in Figure 1, is comprised of a cell body, and extensions from the cell body, the dendrites and the axon. Structures like nucleus, endoplasmic reticulum, golgi apparatus and mitochondria lie in the cell body of the neuron. Neuron is connected to other neurons via dendrites extending from the axons.

The dendrite is the region involved with the reception of the information and the stimuli, and direction of those to the cell body, whereas the cell body is the site of information processing, and the axon and apical part of the axon are the regions of information transmission to other neurons. The cell body is responsible from all activities necessary for its survival (Minneman, 1991). Dendrites are also called the "afferent fibers". Axons carry the received information away from the cell body. Axons are also called the "efferent fibers". Neuron cell bodies form the gray matter in brain and medulla spinalis, and rest of the neurons form the white matter (Uzbay, 2004).

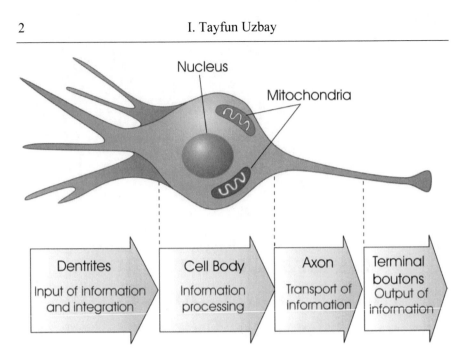

Figure 1. Structure of the neuron.

Neurons are cells, which gather internal and external stimuli, analyze those stimuli and give a response accordingly, this way neurons contribute to the adaptation of the organism to internal and external environment. Neurons also can themselves generate impulses, like myocardial cells. Until recently, neurons were believed to reach a certain amount in number following birth and decrease with age, and were also believed to be the only group of cells which doesn't have the repair capacity in case of structural damage or degeneration. Today, these beliefs have lost their scientific validity. Especially in the hippocampus of rat and human, neurons were shown to be able to regenerate, and new neuron formation was also shown (Erickson et al, 1998; McKim, 2000). Nowadays, not only degenerative diseases like Parkinson's and Alzheimer's disease, but also depression are proposed to result from degeneration of especially hippocampal neurons, and there are some evidences suggesting that antidepressants act through prevention of neuronal degeneration as well as genesis of healthy new neurons (Vogel, 2000, Czeh et al, 2001; Duman, 2002). These evidences strengthen the idea that neurons can regenerate themselves, like other cells in human body.

Concept of Synapse and Neurochemical Transmission

In order for the living organism to adapt the internal and external environment, signals from those sources should be received, transmitted from one neuron to another, modified, evaluated, and stored, if necessary. All these processes take place through neuronal junctions present in the nervous system. Synapse is the principal region in those junctions, where the stimulus or the information is transmitted. Synapse has three compartments morphologically: presynaptic terminal, synaptic cleft and postsynaptic area (Brown and McKim, 2000; Uzbay, 2004) (Figure 2).

Axons approaching to the cell membrane targeted for signal transmission (postsynaptic membrane), branch into less than 1 micron thick extensions. These extensions become rounded as they approach to the postsynaptic membrane and form button like expansions, which are called presynaptic terminals (Figure 2). Neurotransmitters, which are chemical transmitters synthesized in the neurons, are stored in those terminals in "vesicles". During the neurotransmitter release process, these vesicles approach to the presynaptic membrane and open releasing the neurotransmitter into the synaptic cleft (Uzbay, 2004) (Figure 2).

Postsynaptic area is the place where the neuronal signals are transmitted or received. In synapses between two neurons, postsynaptic area is usually on the dendrites of the receptive neuron. Any effector cell (like muscle cells or glandular cells) in contact with the neuron can also form the postsynaptic area.

The dendrites receiving the stimulus or the effector cell membrane is called the postsynaptic membrane. Postsynaptic membrane is approximately 70 angstron thick and has the lipid-protein-lipid structure. On this membrane lie the receptors which are proteins binding the chemical transmitters (neurotransmitters) released from the presynaptic membrane (Uzbay, 2004) (Figure 2).

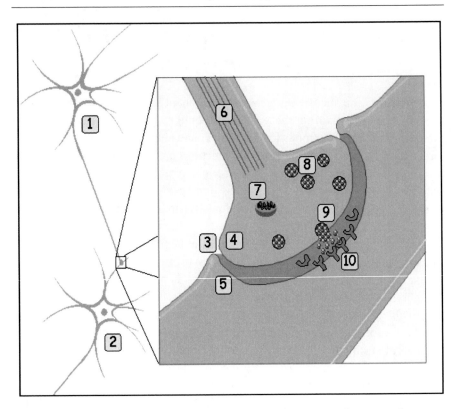

Figure 2. Morphology of synapse. 1: presynaptic neuron, 2: postsynaptic neurons, 3: synaptic cleft, 4: presynaptic terminal, 5: postsynaptic region, 6: microtubules, 7: mitochondria, 8: vesicles storing meurotransmitter, 9: neurotransmitter released from the presynaptic vesicle into the synaptic cleft, 10: receptors on postsynaptic membrane (Uzbay, 2004).

Synaptic cleft is the approximately 250 angstron long gap between the presynaptic and postsynaptic membranes. Neurotransmitters released from the presynaptic terminal, cross the cleft via diffusion, and bind their specific receptors on postsynaptic membrane. Following this, neurotransmitters interact in a specific manner with the protein structures on the postsynaptic membrane, which are called the receptors; this way they transmit the stimulus or the neuronal impulse. As a result, receptive (postsynaptic) cell responds according to the quality of the impulse (Mann and Brown, 1985; Brown and McKim, 2000; Uzbay, 2004) . This sequence of events, which is called neurochemical transmission, is the basic process of central nervous system. The behavior of the species in which a nervous system is developed also depends on the neurochemical transmission. Functioning level of this transmission plays important roles in the pathophysiology and pharmacotherapy of many disorders of nervous system.

Postsynaptic receptors can be conceptualized as detectors which constantly sense the existence of chemicals specific to them, and bind when they found any. Neurotransmitter-receptor binding is formed via electrostatic bonds. The receptor is inactive in the absence of agonists (transmitters, drug molecules or other endogenous molecules which can bind the receptor). The catalytic enzymes present in the postsynaptic membranes play a role in the mediation of the effects of receptors on postsynaptic area. Best known of those catalytic enzymes are "adenylate cyclase", "guanylate cyclase", "phospholipase C" and "phospholipase A2". There are also regulatory proteins in the postsynaptic membrane which regulate the interaction between the catalytic enzymes and the receptors. These proteins are called G proteins. Postsynaptic receptors are localised on the external surface of the membrane. The catalytic enzymes and the regulatory proteins which interact with the receptors lie on the inner surface of the membrane. Initially, chemical transmitter and the receptor form the transmitter-receptor complex. As a result of this interaction, membrane fluidity increases, and the complex approaches to the regulatory proteins and the catalytic enzymes. Then, transmitter-receptor-G protein complex is formed. Depending on the quality of the G protein in the complex, this interaction results in activation or inhibition of the adenylate cyclase. This may increase or decrease intracellular synthesis of cyclic adenosine monophosphate (cAMP), respectively. If the G protein in the complex is stimulatory (Gs) synthesis increases, if it is inhibitory (Gi), synthesis decreases. There are other types of G proteins playing important roles in intracellular biological processes. The synthesis of cAMP triggers the cascade of events in the neuron which result in emergence of the biological end response (Minneman, 1991; Ozawa et al, 1998).

Transmitters, drug molecules or endogenous molecules, act as primary messengers as they convey the biological stimulus to the cytoplasm. Other mediators in the cytoplasm, act as second messengers, further carrying the signal. The cyclic nucleotides, cAMP and cyclic guanosine monophosphate (cGMP), are important elements of second messengers. Besides, Ca/calmodulin that activates protein kinases, arachidonic acid, inositol triphosphate and diacylglycerol act as second messangers in the transmission of the biological signals (Minneman, 1991; Ozawa et al, 1998).

Neurotransmitters and Gene Regulation

The changes in transcription of genes may result in change in rates of synthesis of some cellular proteins, or disruption of the structure of the proteins. There is increasing evidence indicating that neurotransmitters mediating the neurochemical transmission via being released to the synaptic cleft, can regulate gene expression in the nucleus in a similar way. Gene expression has an important contribution to the adaptive responses in long term, in response to the drugs and external factors (Feldman et al, 1997; McKim, 2000).

The activation of genes occurs in two steps. Gene activation always starts with a synaptic stimulus (Armstrong and Montminy, 1993). The initiation phase, which is the first step in gene activation, occurs with the stimulation of "immediate early genes" (IEG). IEGs are in low levels when there is no cellular excitation. With the activation of synaptic input (stimulus), IEGs are induced rapidly and transiently. For example, levels of mRNA are increased significantly in 15 minutes. This increase is not permanent and persists only for 30-60 minutes. In the second step, "late initiation genes" (LIG) are activated. Since the activation of these genes depends on the activation of IEGs, their response is slower.

Substances madiating the neurochemical transmission in the synaptic cleft can regulate the gene expression, with a complex mechanism, with the contribution of "transription factors" and second messengers like cAMP, cGMP, and Ca^{2+}. Second messengers work together with some transcription factors in cases in which the neurotransmitters have a role in gene expression. For example, in the activation of the transcription via cAMP, a short segment of DNA, including 8 nucleotides, is involved, this region is called "cAMP response element" (CRE). Initially, cAMP is synthesized and activates intracellular "protein kinase A" (PKA). Following activation, catalytic subunits of PKA, are transferred into the nucleus (translocation), and here phosphorylate a nuclear protein, called CRE binding protein (CREB) (Vallejo, 1994). CREB acts as a transcription factor and mediates gene transcription. CREB can be phosphorylated with some other kinases besides PKA.

c-fos is another IEG, and is also a proto-oncogene. The transcription factor coded with c-fos is called Fos. It was shown with immunohistochemistry that Fos and c-fos mRNA are present in the brain. Like in other IEGs, levels of Fos and c-fos mRNA are low when there is no stimulation. Excitation of the neuron with the binding of a neurotransmitter to a receptor on the postsynaptic membrane increases second messengers like cAMP and Ca.

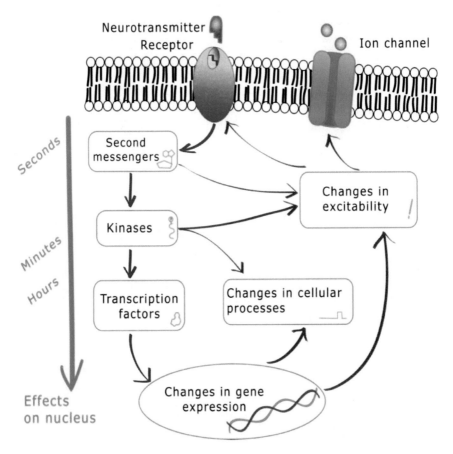

Figure 3. Gene expression through neurotransmission in the central nervous system.

The increase in the second messengers rapidly induces Fos expression, through CREB and some other transcription factors. The factor stimulating the neuron can as well be an external factor or a pharmacological factor like a drug molecule. In this case, c-fos and other IEGs serve as an indicator of neuronal activation (Morgan and Curran, 1989; Sagar and Sharp, 1993). It has been suggested that IEGs play an important role in central nervous system plasticity, and learning which is a type of plasticity (Abraham et al, 1991). Fos expression, since it is sensitive to various drugs, is of special interest to the neuropharmacologs. There are reports of fos induction in some brain regions in response to caffein (Nakajima et al, 1989), amphetamine and cocaine

(Graybiel et al, 1990), haloperidol adn some other neuroleptics (Dragunow et al, 1990), morphine (Liu et al, 1994), nicotine (Kiba and Jayaraman, 1994), and tetrahydrocannabinol -the active chemical in cannabis- (Mailleux et al, 1994). It has been proposed that, in striatum, CREB phosphorylation via dopamine D1 receptor plays an important role in Fos response to amphetamine (Konradi et al, 1994). Fos and other IEGs are important elements which can help in exploration of the mechanisms of regulation of gene expression in the cenral nervous system through drugs and neurotransmitters. Gene expression in the central nervous system with neurotransmitters is presented in short in figure 3; and resulting plasticity is shown in Figure 4 in the example of noradrenaline and serotonine.

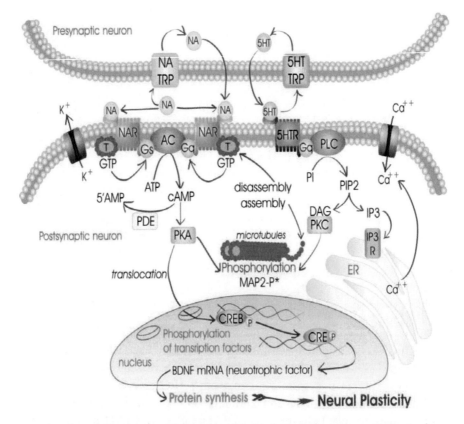

Figure 4. Gene expression through neurotransmission in the central nervous system and neuroplasticity (NA: noradrenaline, 5-HT: serotonine, AC: adenylate cyclase, PLC: phospholipase C, PKC: phosphokinase C, DAG: diacylglicerol, IP3: inositol triphosphate; Gs, Gi, and Gq: stimulator, inhibitor and q type G proteins, respectively, CREB: cAMP response element binding protein.

Principal Neuroanatomical Regions in the Central Nervous System with Functional Importance

Cerebral cortex, limbic system, diencephalon, mesencephalon, serebellum, brain stem and medulla spinalis are the principal regions in central nervous system (Figure 5). These regions and structures located within them, like medulla, reticular activating system, locus ceruleus, basal ganglia and periaquaductal grey matter reponsible from all affects and behaviors in sophisticated living things (Minneman, 1991; Brick and Erickson, 1998; McKim, 2000).

Spinal cord serves as a relay station for the integration of the information and execution of reflex activities. It conveys information coming from sensory neurons and conveys motor commands from brain to the muscles. The central part of the spinal cord is called grey matter. The axons of the sensory neurons enter into the grey matter in spinal cord from the dorsal side, and motor fibers leave the cord from the ventral side. The ventral horn of the grey matter in spinal cord contains cell bodies of the motor neurons; these neurons are directly related to muscular activity. This region is also important in formation of many reflexes. Dorsal horn also contains neurons which transmit sensory information.

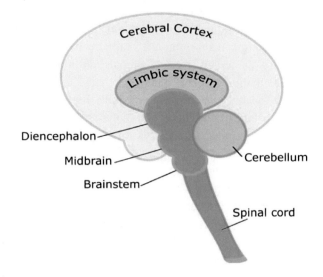

Figure 5. Principle neuroanatomic regions in central nervous system.

Medulla is the region lying in the base of the brain and brain stem. It begins immediately after the spinal cord. Many neurons related to autonomic nervous system enter in and exit from the brain through medulla. In medulla there are some centers related to vital functions. One of these is the respiratory center which controls breathing. Respiratory center in the medulla is sensitive to barbiturates, opiates and alcohol which dose-dependently suppress its activity. Overdose and intoxications with those drugs, results in coma and death due to the suppression of the respiratory center. Another center in this region is the chemoreceptor trigger zone (CTZ) which is responsible from the regulation of nausea and vomitting. CTZ is sensitive to pharmacological agents like opiates and nicotine. Intaking these drugs causes nausea and vomitting via dose-dependently stimulating of CTZ.

Two dense nerve projections originating from the medulla and projecting to higher regions are *"reticular activating system"* (RAS) and *"raphe system"*. One of the most important functions of the RAS is to maintain the cortical activation and control the state of arousal. Drugs which increase the activity of inhibitor neurotransmitters like GABA, depress RAS and arousal. The stimulation of the raphe system is related to the formation of sleep. Raphe nucleus is in the brainstem and serotonine is the major neurotransmitter. Drugs that modulate serotonergic activity in this region also affect sleep. Neuronal axons in the raphe nucleus project to the limbic system and forebrain through medial forebrain bundle and play a role in mood regulation.

Locus ceruleus is another nucleus located in brainstem. Projections from the neurons in locus ceruleus extend to limbic system and cortex. The major neurotransmitter in locus ceruleus is noradrenalin. It is believed that more than half of the noradrenergic neurons in the brain lie in locus ceruleus. Locus ceruleus causes fear, panic and anger in animals and human. This region has important role in formation of anxiety and panic attacks.

Cerebellum is located just above the medulla. Its functions are related to motor system. Voluntary motor action is initiated and controlled via a part of cortex, motor cortex. Serebellum receives direct projections from the motor cortex and muscles through the spinal cord. It is important in formation and regulation of voluntary motor actions. Among other functions mediated by the cerebellum are the eye movements and learning related processes.

Basal ganglia are subcortical nuclei located in the cerebral hemispheres, above the brain stem and in the grey matter. Anatomically it contains "caudate nucleus", "putamen", "globus pallidus", "amygdaloid complex". Globus pallidus and putamen together are also called "lenticular nucleus". And, lenticular nucleus and caudate nucleus are together called "corpus striatum".

Putamen and caudate nucleus together are called "striatum". Striatum mainly receives projections from cerebral cortex and thalamus, and axons extend to globus pallidum. Striatum is the input area for the neuronal fibers to the basal ganglia, and globus pallidum is the output area. Basal ganglia have an essantial role in regulation of voluntary motor activity. Lesions in basal ganglia, results in diseases characterised with movement system problems, like Parkinson disease. Basal ganglia also have contribuiton to the regulation of eyemovements and spatial memory.

Periaquaductal grey matter (PGM) is a structure functioning along the cenral part of the brain. It contributes to two important functions of the central nervous system. These are the perception of pain and aversive stimuli. PGM acts as a relay station for the axons carrying noxious stimuli from the dorsal horn of the spinal cord. This region is rich in opioid receptors. Electrical stimulaiton of the PGM in animals causes the perception, differentiation and learning of the aversive stimuli.

Limbic system is mainly responsible from the regulation of mood and motivation. It contains hypothalamus, nucleus accumbens, hippocampus, amygdala, and septum. Lesions of some parts of hypothalamus may result in excessive increase or abolishing of eating and drinking behaviour in animals. Food related reinforcement in animals is believed to be mediated through hypothalamus. Mesolimbic dopaminergic system is formed by the projections from the ventral tegmental area of the midbrain to the limbic system (particularly to nucleus accumbens); and it is responsible from reward. Dysfunctions in this system may be responsible from schizophrenia.

Hippocampus is a limbic structure especially related to memory and learning. Many years before surgical removal or lesioning of hippocampus as a treatment of epilepsy, were reported to result in serious amnesia. In rats, hippocampus is closely related to spatial memory, and lesions may cause deficits in learning and memory.

Amygdala and *septum* are other two limbic structures receiving serotonergic projections from the raphe nucleus. Amygdala is especially related to formation of anxiety and aggression. Lesioning of this region abolishes aggression and anxiety, whereas electrical stimulation causes excessive increase in these behaviours in animals. Lesions of septum in laboratory animals result in changes in affect.

Cerebral cortex is the highest and most complex part of the brain. Glutamate and GABA are the two main neurotransmitters, excitatory and inhibitory, respectively. The most important function of the cortex is the management of integration of the sensory information received from lower centers. It has important contribution to the regulation of motor activity. It has specialised parts for the recognition of spoken or written language. Besides, more importantly, it has important role in the formation of mental processes related with cognition and thoughts.

Chapter 2

Mental Diseases, the Contribution of Stress and Hippocampal Disorders

Hippocampus: Neuroanatomy, Histology and Hippocampal Neural Pathways

Hippocampus is the most important region in the brain about neuroplasticity. There may be two reasons for this. First, it is really rich in incoming and outgoing fibers (Figure 6), and is densely connected to other parts of the limbic system, especially amygdala. Second, it is the center for basic adaptive responses: memory and learning.

Thus, due to the main subject of this book, we will be reviewing neuroanatomy, neurohistology of hippocampus and stress related changes in hippocampus in more detail. Hippocampus is an important neuroanatomic structure in midbrain limbic system (Figure 7).

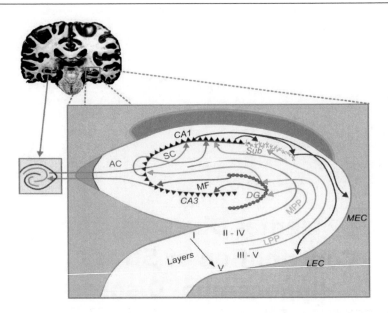

Figure 6. Hippocampal neural circuits. Nerve fibers coming to hippocampus from lateral and medial entorhinal cortex (LEC, MEC) are connected to pyramidal neurons in CA3 region of cornu ammonis (CA) and dentate gyrus (DG) through perforant pathway. CA3 neurons receive neural input from DG through mossy fibers (MF), and project their axons over Schaffer collaterals (SC) and commissural pathway to CA1 regions. CA1 neurons receive direct fibers form perforant pathway and project axons to subiculum. Fibers starting from this region project back to entorhinal cortex forming the hippocampal output.

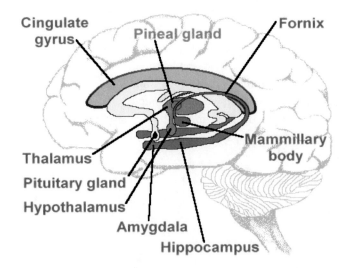

Figure 7. Hippocampus and limbic system.

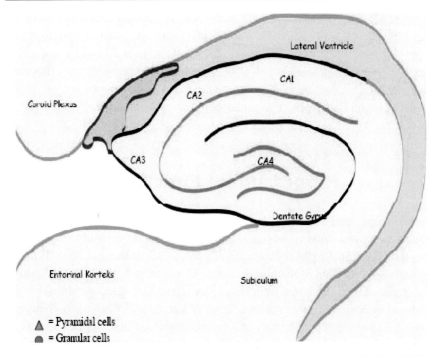

Figure 8. Neuroanatomical subregions of hippocampus in a coronal section (Uzbay, 2005).

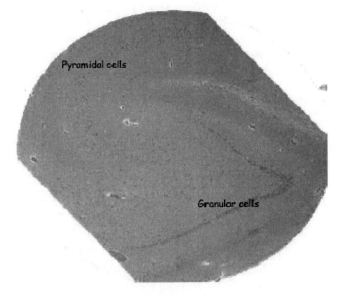

Figure 9. Microscopic appearance of pyramidal cells in cornu ammonis and granular cells in dentate gyrus, in the hippocampus (Uzbay, 2005).

Hippocampus is circumvented with lateral ventricule, entorhinal cortex and subiculum. Cornu ammonis and dentate gyrus are the functionally most important parts of the hippocampus (Figure 8). Cornu ammonis can be divided into 4 subregions, named CA1 to CA4. Pyramidal and granular cells that may easily be seen with microscopic examination are the most important functional elements of hippocampus. Pyramidal cells are distributed from the CA1 to CA4, wheras granular cells are localised to dentate gyrus (Figure 8, 9).

Hippocampal Functions

In human and laboratory animals, hippocampus has important role in physiologic processes relevant to learning and memory formation. "Septohippocampal pathway", originating from the cholinergic neurons in the septum and projecting to the hippocampus, is related to learning and regulation and management of short-term memeory functions. Degeneration of the cholinergic neurons causes various forms of demantia, including Alzheimer's disease. Many studies on human and animals conclude that hippocampus is an important brain region involved in memory formation (Squire, 1992; Sala et al, 2004). Together with amygdala and orbitofrontal cortex, hippocampus has important contribution in information processing and formation of declarative memory (Poldrack and Gabrieli, 1997; Shu et al, 2003). It is known that, emotional memory is formed in amygdala (Cahill, 2000), and declarative memory formation, including cases with verbal expression occurs in hippocampus (Brewin, 2001). Hippocampus is also important in "memory consolidation" which is the process of conversion of short-term memory to long-term memory in the neocortex. Here, hippocampus plays a critical role in supplying the first input necessary for the long-term memory, conversion of these to long-term memories, and formation and strenghtening of the synaptic connections necessary for the maintenance of long-term memory (Wittenberg and Tsien, 2002; Sala et al, 2004).

Hippocampus, working together with amygdala, is related to conditioned fear response. A stimulus that may cause fear and threat reaches to amygdala, which is the most imporant structure about these emotions; hippocampus and some other cortical structures are also stimulated independent from amygdala. Hippocampus performs the necessary function of processing and realisation of the stimulus (Sala et al, 2004). This immediately leads to better interpretation of the fearful stimulus and evaluation of the real threatening value, initiation of the memory processes necessary for taking precautions, and neglecting the stimulus if it is not a real threat. Improper functioning of the hippocampus, results in the incapability of the organism in rationally responding to the stimuli. This condition may be related to many psychiatric problems, like anxiety and suicide.

There are two stages in the process of stress related disorders. First, there is an increase in catecholaminergic activity and because of that there is an increase in amount and rate of flow of oxygen and glucose into the brain. This is a beneficial condition, in that it results in an acute increase in cognitive processes with the stimulus. This can be an example of the organism's increasing level of arousal in case of a threatening situation. Still, prolonged duration of exposure to the increased levels of catecholamines may interfere with the cognitive functions (McEwen and Sapolsky, 1995). In the second stage, HPA is stimulated in response to the stres, resulting in increased glucocorticoid release and levels. Increased levels of glucocorticoids can supress learning related neuronal processes like "long term potentiation" (LTP) in hippocampus (Sala et al, 2004). Low levels of glucocorticoids enhance neuronal processes like LTP, wheras higher levels supress. This data has been consistently proven to be true with many experiments (Diamond and Rose, 1994; McEwen and Sapolsky, 1995; Pavlides et al, 1995; Lupien and McEwen, 1997).

Another important function of hippocampus is the regulation of response to stress. It is not yet clearly known which neurotransmitter systems are involved in the regulation of responses during and after repetitive distressing stimuli in the hippocampus. Though there are clear evidences that glucocorticoids, particularly corticosterone, and excitatory aminoacids, particularly glutamate have significant contributions. Glucocorticoids are believed to act in collaboration with excitatory aminoacids, serotonine and GABA in the regulation of these responses (Sala et al, 2004).

In laboratory animals, with the first exposure to stress, there is an increase in glutamate release in prefrontal cortex and prefrontal areas; this causes increase of monoamines in brain regions like ventral striatum, amygdala and prefrontal areas (Moghaddam, 2002). Within these conditions, hippocampus regulates the activity of hypothalamohypophysealadrenal axis (HPA) through its projections to the neuroendocrine related areas of the paraventricular nuclei. In the studies of stress reactions of animals, it was suggested that increased levels of glucocorticoids decrease the capacity of hippocampus to supress HPA, and this resulted in the hypothesis of "glucocorticoid turnover". According to this hypothesis, excessive stress or glucocorticoid use damages the hippocampus and cause severe injury. This hypothesis received important support from findings of some preclinical studies (McEwen 1999a, b; Sapolsky, 2000; Sala, 2004). In several species of laboratory animals, it is shown that there may be a correlation between increased levels of glucocorticoids during distress and structural damage in the hippocampus (Uno et al, 1989; Sapolsky et al, 1990; Watanabe et al, 1992). In several studies in which high levels of glucocorticoids are applied for prolonged periods or restrain stress was applied, it has been shown that significant level of damage at cellular level occur, like increased neuronal dendritic reshaping (Woolley et al, 1990), apical atrophy in the dendrites (Magarinos et al, 1996; Watanabe et al, 1992), structural changes in synapses (Magarinos et al, 1997), suppression of neurogenesis (Gould et al, 1998; Duman et al, 2001), increase of neuronal loss (Uno et al, 1989, Mizoguchi et al, 1992), in the hippocampus.

Glucocorticoids applied exogenously, or released in increased amounts in response to the stress, increase glutamatergic activity in the hippocampus (Moghaddam et al, 1994; 2002; Stein-Behrens et al, 1994; Venero and Borrel, 1999). High levels of glutamate have disadvantageous effects on the hippocampus due to stimulation of NMDA receptors and increase in intracellular Ca (Landfield, 1994). Both inhibitors of steroid synthesis and NMDA receptor antagonists were shown to repair the dendritic atrophy caused by stress (Magarinos and McEwen, 1995a, b). These observations indicate that high levels of glucocorticoids released as a response to stress, can result in severe damage in hippocampus, through increasing inflow of Ca via stimulation of NMDA receptors.

It can be assumed that, serotonine has a role in stress-induced damage in the hippocampus due. It is reported that serotonine release is increased during stress (Chaouloff, 1993). There are studies indicating that the damage in the CA3 region of the hippocampus resulting from stress can be prevented by application of tianeptin, an antidepressant increasing serotonine reuptake (Watanabe et al, 1992; McEwen et al, 1997; Magarinos et al, 1999). Findings of these studies support that hypothesis. There is not still enough evidence to consider that serotonine or serotonergic system have as strong influence in the stress response in hippocampus as glutamate has. Yet, it is not clearly known how tianeptin affects the serotonergic system (Pineyro and blier, 1999), and there is the possibility that it may have positive effects on the hippocampal injury due to the interaction with other neurotransmitter system. Recent studies have shown that tianeptin blocks free radical nitric oxide (Wegener et al, 2003), which is known to cause neuronal injury and excitatory responses activating the glutamatergic system in the central nervous system (Garthwaite,

1991; Uzbay and Oglesby, 2001), and it directly inhibits glutamatergic activity in hippocampus (Kole et al, 2002; Reagan et al, 2004). The effects of tianeptin on the stress related damage in hippocampus and probable mechanisms of action will be explored in greater detail in later sections of this book.

There are many publications indicating that stress induced changes in hippocampus can be related to psychiatric disorders like posttraumatic stress disorder, borderline personality disorder and depression. Hippocampal changes in depression and relevance of stress induced changes in hippocampus and depression will be discussed later in this book, under the title of neuroplasticity.

Chapter 3

Depression and Neurobiology of Depression

Depression is an important psychiatric disorder that affects individuals' quality of life and social relations directly. Depression is characterized by emotional symptoms such as hopelessness, apathy, loss of self-confidence, sense of guilt, indecisiveness, and amotivation, as well as biological symptoms like psychomotor retardation, loss of libido, sleep disturbances, and loss of appetite. When the symptoms are very severe major depression is considered. The prevalence of major depression is approximately 9% in both the United States and Europe (Fichter et al, 1996; Lepine et al, 1997).

Depression should be considered a disease to be definitely followed and treated because of its prevalence, negative effect on the workforce, and suicidal outcome. However, depression is underdiagnosed for several reasons (Richelson, 2001).

One of the main reasons is the lack of objective diagnostic methods like neuroimaging techniques. Today the diagnosis of depression also depends on the information obtained from the patient and assessment of this information in the context of several scales. These assessments occasionally yield false or insufficient diagnoses due to the subjectivity of the data.

In recent years, the contribution of pharmacotherapy to depression treatment has become greater. Depression treatment mostly requires long-term, chronic antidepressant therapy, and thus the side effects and safety of available antidepressants are of great importance. A substantial proportion of the adverse effects of antidepressants are explained by their synaptic effects.

Changes in the synaptic activity of many neurotransmitters, especially serotonin and noradrenalin, due to these drugs account for many of these side effects as well as their antidepressant activity (Richelson, 2001). The neurobiological mechanisms underlying depression should be clarified in order to diagnose depression more reliably and to treat it more effectively by developing more specific drugs.

Today, the most widely accepted opinion about depression concerns its direct relation with noradrenergic and serotonergic systems. The mechanism of action of available antidepressants involves one or both of these systems. Therefore, a general overview of noradrenergic and serotonergic systems will also be included in this section.

Noradrenergic System

Many of the adrenergic neuron bodies are located at a nucleus in the brainstem, namely the locus ceruleus (LC). This is a center that also executes other functions like behavior, cognition, mood, emotions, and movements. Noradrenergic fibers originating from the LC join to the medial forebrain bundle and form projections to the limbic system, hypothalamus, and cortex (Figure 10).

The noradrenergic system is responsible for the modulation of arousal, modulation of mood, and central modulation of blood pressure and heart rate. Increased noradrenergic activity is associated with anxiety, mania, hypervigilance, and induction of the brain reward system. Decreased noradrenergic activity is known to be associated with depression as well as decreased attention and concentration, impairment in working memory, slowed information processing, psychomotor retardation and fatigue (Stahl, 1996).

Decreased noradrenergic transmission is proposed to contribute to some schizophrenic symptoms (Bird et al, 1979; Snyder, 1982). Noradrenalin contributes to the motor effects of dopamine. In Parkinson's disease decreased noradrenergic activity due to noradrenergic neuron damage in the brainstem also contributes to motor impairment although not as much as the dopamine system does (Marsden, 1982). Noradrenergic neuron destruction also contributes to the symptoms in Alzheimer's disease due to a cholinergic defect.

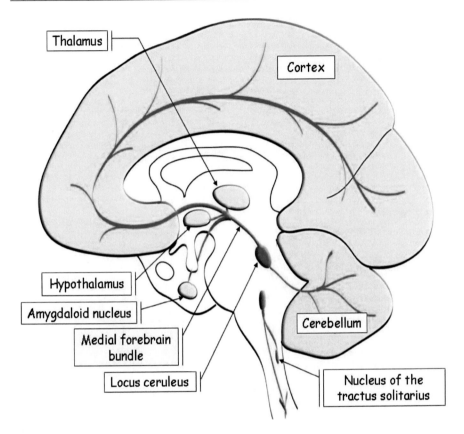

Figure 10. Brain noradrenergic system (Uzbay, 2004).

Serotonergic System

Serotonin is a neurotransmitter in the central nervous system and a transmitter that has neuromodulatory effects on different effector cells at the periphery. Neurons localized in the brainstem dorsal and median raphe nuclei are the primary sources of serotonin (Ninan, 1999). Serotonergic fibers originating from the raphe nucleus form projections to the thalamus, hypothalamus, limbic system, striatum, cerebral cortex and cerebellum (Figure 11).

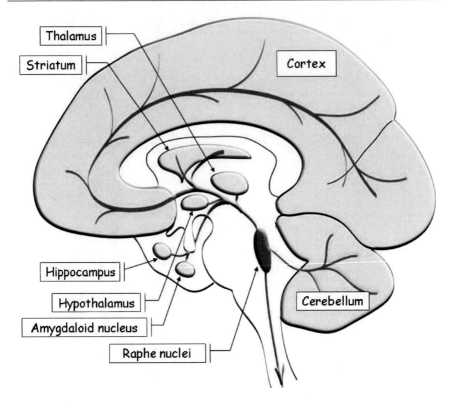

Figure 11. Brain serotonergic system (Uzbay, 2004).

The main functions of the serotonergic system in the central nervous system are listed below.

Mood

The role of serotonin in anxiety is supported by its modulatory effects over the LC and by serotonergic fibers reaching the amygdala (Dubovsky and Thomas, 1995; Ninan, 1999).

The interaction between serotonergic and noradrenergic systems may be associated with anxiety development. Research on monkey brains shows that the LC has serotonergic neurons as well as noradrenergic neurons. In addition, the brainstem raphe system, which may be regarded as the central serotonergic center, is also innervated by noradrenergic neurons and the LC receives serotonergic innervation from the brainstem raphe system (Mason and Fibiger,

1979; Hohen-Saric, 1982; Ninan, 1999). It is proposed that modulation of central serotonergic activity has a role in the anxiolytic effects of benzodiazepines besides their interaction with the LC and the noradrenergic system (Stein et al, 1975; Sepinwall and Cook, 1980). Important data indicate that among the serotonin receptors presynaptic 5-HT1A autoreceptors and postsynaptic 5-HT3 receptors are associated with anxiety. 5-HT1A receptor agonist drugs such as buspiron, ipsapiron and gepiron are used in the treatment of generalized anxiety disorder in particular (Goldberg and Finnerty, 1979; Yocca, 1990). It is also observed that serotonin 5-HT3 receptor blockage has positive effects in several experimental anxiety models.

These findings suggest that 5-HT3 receptor antagonists like ondansetron may be a novel class of drugs for anxiety treatment (Rang et al, 1998; Olivier et al, 2000). Recently, selective serotonin reuptake inhibitors like fluoxetine and noradrenalin and serotonin reuptake inhibitors like venlafaxin have been observed to be effective in the treatment of different anxiety disorders (Stahl, 1996; Rang et al, 1999, Allgulander et al, 2001). However, the mechanism of action of these antidepressants on serotonin and noradrenalin in the treatment of anxiety has not been clearly identified yet.

A decrease in serotonergic activity is associated with depression. In experimental studies decreases in brain serotonergic activity due to social isolation have been known about for a long time (Garattini et al, 1967).

Specifically, rodents display hyperactive and aggressive behavior during long-term social isolation that can be blocked with antidepressant treatment (Garzon and del Rio, 1981). These social isolation forms based on serotonin deficiency are used as experimental depression models in rodents (Leonard, 1998). On the other hand, selective serotonin reuptake inhibitors and some postsynaptic receptor agonists who increase serotonergic activity in the synaptic space, are used widely and effectively for treating depression (Cowen, 1998; Vaswani et al, 2003).

Hallucinations and Behavioral Changes

Serotonin analogues like LSD depress brainstem serotonergic neurons that are responsible for inhibition in the cortical area. This loss of inhibition is thought to be responsible for hallucinogenic effects. Serotonin precursors cause 'wet dog shake' behavior in experimental animals (Rang et al, 1999).

Modulation of Sleep and Arousal

Degeneration of the raphe nucleus and serotonergic hypoactivity inhibit sleep, and serotonin microinjection to the brainstem induces sleep (Rang et al, 1999).

Nociception

Serotonin has inhibitory effects on pain conductance in the spinal channel. Depletion of serotonin via parachlorphenylalanine (pCPA) or selective lesions of serotonin containing descending neurons inhibits the analgesic effects of morphine in experimental animals (Uzbay et al, 1999).

Modulation of Eating and Drinking Behavior

Serotonergic drugs in the paraventricular nucleus of the hypothalamus contribute to the control of appetite. Anticholinergic drugs may cause weight gain by increasing appetite (Rang et al, 1999).

Other

5-HT3 receptor antagonists like ondansetron have strong antiemetic effects. They inhibit nausea and vomiting, particularly during chemotherapy. Serotonin is also associated with temperature regulation and sexual dysfunction (Rang et al, 1999).

Monoamine Hypothesis of Depression

Most information about the mechanism of depression depends on the monoamine hypothesis, which is still partially valid today. The main biochemical hypothesis proposed in depression is based on a direct relationship between the occurrence of depression and loss of monoamine neurotransmitters, especially noradrenalin and serotonin, in certain areas of the brain (Bunney and Davis, 1965; Schildkraut, 1965). In mania there is hyperfunction of these neurotransmitters in the same regions. This hypothesis is supported by the depression-treating effects of drugs like tricyclic antidepressants, monoamine oxidase inhibitors and selective serotonin reuptake inhibitors (SSRI) that increase monoaminergic transmission and effectiveness in synapses in contrast to the depression-causing effect of reserpine, a drug that has activity opposite to these drugs, in both humans and animals (Leonard, 1998; Delgado et al, 1998).

In biochemical studies of depressive patients, although not in all forms of depression, results supporting monoamine hypothesis were obtained in many patients (Bondy, 2002). The contribution of noradrenalin to depression is confirmed by the observation of significantly decreased renal excretion of its metabolite 3-methoxy-4-hydroxyphenylglycol (MHPG) in depressive patients compared with normal controls (Maas et al, 1968). Serotonin's role in depression has been subject to more detailed studies, and the view that serotonin is the major monoamine associated with the development of depression has gained importance over time. In studies, amounts of 5-hydroxyindol acetic acid (5-HIAA), the major metabolite of serotonin, in cerebrospinal fluid, and tryptophan, the free precursor of serotonin in plasma, are found to be lower in depressive patients than in controls (van Praag, 1982a).

Results of postmortem examinations also show that serotonin and serotonin metabolites are significantly lower in several regions of the brain in depressive people (van Praag, 1982b). The most important data proving the importance of biogenic amines concern the antidepressant activity of drugs that increase monoamine activity in the synaptic space by inhibiting monoamine reuptake (tricyclic antidepressants) and enzymatic catabolism (MAO inhibitors).

In line with the monoamine hypothesis, predicting that drugs that increase the synaptic effectiveness of monoamines have antidepressant effects, many drug groups like tricyclic antidepressants and serotonin/noradrenalin reuptake inhibitors (SNRI) have been discovered and used for treatment.

Tricyclics started to be used in the late fifties as the first antidepressants. In this period, based on the opinion that increasing monoamine levels may be successful in depression treatment, monoamine oxidase (MAO) enzyme inhibitors were started to be used along with tricyclic antidepressants. In the sixties and seventies inhibitors specific to MAO subtypes as well as inhibitors specific to noradrenalin and serotonin reuptake started to be used. The main reason for developing more specific drugs is to minimize side effects and to produce a stronger effect. In recent years drugs that are more specific to one of these monoamines like selective serotonin reuptake inhibitors such as fluoxetine and paroxetine and selective noradrenalin reuptake inhibitors such as reboxetine have become part of antidepressant treatment (Pacher et al, 2001).

Studies on drugs that affect the serotonin system were not limited to serotonin reuptake inhibition in the synaptic space. Attempts were made to develop other drugs affecting serotonin receptors, especially 5-HT2 and 5-HT3, and these drugs are widely used in depression treatment (Hindmarch, 2002; Kennedy et al, 2004).

Is the Monoamine Hypothesis Alone Sufficient to Explain Depression?

Whether monoamine hypothesis can explain all parameters associated with depression has been discussed for a long time. There are two important problems regarding the monoamine hypothesis. The first is the presence of refractory depression cases that do not respond to any antidepressant. Their number is too high to be neglected. The second important and interesting problem is the antidepressant effects of some drugs that have opposite effects on monoamines and the lack of significant differences between the antidepressant effects of these drugs.

The most interesting example of this is the similar antidepressant effectiveness of tianeptine, a drug defined as an atypical antidepressant by some authors, and SSRIs, which have a theoretically opposite mechanism of action. The addition of tianeptine to antidepressant treatment led to a debate on the serotonin part of the monoamine hypothesis and forced scientists to seek new insights.

The tianeptine molecule was synthesized at the Servier Institute, France, at the beginning of the eighties during research to develop new antidepressant drugs more effective and safer than tricyclics. Its molecular formulation is $C_{21}H_{24}ClN_2NaO_4S$, and its molecular structure includes a substituted dibenzotiazepine nucleus and a long aminoheptanoic acid side chain (figure 12). This 7 carbon amino acid ($NH-(CH_2)_6-COONa$) side chain distinguishes it from tricyclic antidepressants.

Tianeptine is an antidepressant primarily acting on the serotonergic system. It does not inhibit serotonin reuptake as many antidepressants do; instead it increases serotonin reuptake selectively in both the brain and thrombocytes. This effect occurs after both acute and chronic administration (Menini et al, 1987; Kato and Weitsch, 1988; Fattacini et al, 1990).

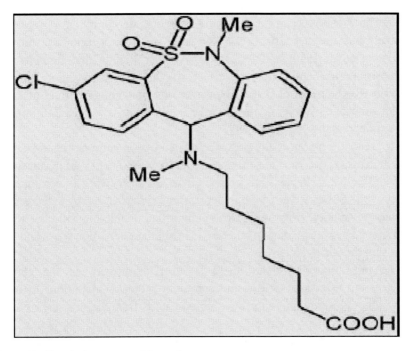

Figure 12. Chemical structure of tianeptine.

In contrast to tricyclic antidepressants and SSRIs, tianeptine decreases serotonin's activity and amount in serotonergic synapses of the central nervous system by increasing serotonin reuptake. The antidepressant effects and similar antidepressant effectiveness of tianeptine, and SSRIs that have opposite mechanisms of action on the serotonergic system (Loo et al, 1999; Waintraub et al, 2000) are an interesting point indicating that central mechanisms of action associated with depression should be reviewed. The following opinions attempt to explain the antidepressant effectiveness of tianeptine (Ansseau, 1993; Uzbay and Yüksel, 2002).

The first hypothesis states that diseases may be characterized more by increases in serotonergic neurotransmission than by serotonin decreases, and therefore agents decreasing serotonin levels have good antidepressant effectiveness. Indeed, it is reported that many antidepressant drugs can cause a degree of 5-HT receptor blockage, and receptor blocking effects may be dominant over serotonergic activity increasing effects. This opinion also suggests the depression hypothesis based on increased serotonergic activity due to several reasons (Aprison et al, 1982). Some antidepressants prominently block post-synaptic 5-HT2 receptors. For example, amitriptilin causes a strong blockage in 5-HT2 receptors while causing moderate inhibition of serotonin reuptake, and the net effect is a decrease in serotonergic transmission (Nagayama et al, 1980; Willner, 1985). Another finding that supports this hypothesis is the antidepressant effect of the 5-HT2 receptor blocker, ritanserin (Reyntjens et al, 1986). However, the predominant effect of 5-HT receptor blockage over serotonin reuptake inhibition is not a general property of all antidepressants (Ansseau, 1993).

The second opinion is the presence of depression subtypes characterized by an increase or decrease in serotonergic activity (Willner, 1985). Tianeptine may be effective in depressions characterized by an increase in serotonergic activity while SSRIs are effective in depressions characterized by a decrease in serotonergic activity. However, placebo-controlled double-blind studies found no difference between tianeptin and SSRIs in similar depression types and thus do not support this hypothesis.

The third opinion is that there is no relation between the clinical antidepressant effects of SSRIs and serotonin reuptake inhibition. In other words, although serotonin reuptake inhibition starts from the first day of SSRI treatment the antidepressant effects of these drugs emerge 2-3 weeks later (Quitkin et al, 1984; Kato and Weitsch, 1998). Moreover, although in vitro and acute administration of classical tricyclics like imipramin and desipramin causes serotonin reuptake inhibition, chronic administration causes serotonin reuptake to increase (Barbaccia et al, 1983). A similar effect is reported for fluvoxamine (Brunello et al, 1987). It is possible to relate these effects of antidepressants with clinical changes following antidepressant treatment. During treatment with serotonin reuptake inhibitors, an increase in depression severity during the first 1-2 weeks followed by a rapid clinical improvement (Ansseau, 1998) may also confirm this opinion. This kind of biphasic clinical change is more common with SSRIs like fluvoxamine (Den Boer and Westenberg, 1998). According to this opinion, tianeptine is an antidepressant drug that produces effects from the beginning of treatment that are produced later by other drugs. No worsening of symptoms with tianeptine at the beginning of antidepressant treatment and a rapid antidepressant effect also support this opinion.

As a result, until the antidepressant effect of tianeptine was shown, it seemed more logical that decreased serotonergic neurotransmission has a role in depression, and the antidepressant effectiveness of SSRIs supported this opinion. Tianeptine, an antidepressant, that has a mechanism of action opposite to that of SSRIs, necessitated a reevaluation of the biochemical basis of depressive disorders and revealed that it cannot be explained solely by the monoamine hypothesis.

An interesting study conducted recently suggests that tianeptine has a mechanism of action similar to that of fluoxetine (Alici et al, 2006). This experimental study examined the drug preference and discrimination producing properties of fluoxetine and tianeptine in rats. The principle of the model used in this test is to overlap the discriminative effects of tianeptine and fluoxetine or the ineffectiveness of saline injections in a mechanism where test subjects may get food using a left or right pedal (Uzbay, 2004). To do this firstly the food intake of the subjects is restricted. Then they are put into cages and stay there for two days to learn to obtain food by pressing a pedal. During the first treatment session the system is adjusted so that the subject receives food when it presses either of the pedals. After the subject learns to get food by pressing a pedal the system is adjusted so that food is given after the subject presses different pedals in response to saline or tianeptine injections. For example, to get food, the subject learns to press the left pedal if saline is injected and the right pedal if tianeptine is injected. After all subjects are taught to differentiate the saline and tianeptine pedals (figure 13) they enter the principle experiment.

During the test the system is adjusted again as the beginning so that food is given if the subject presses either of the pedals. This time fluoxetine is given instead of tianeptin to the subjects that have learned to discriminate between saline and tianeptine. If the substance is tested (fluoxetine) has stimulating properties similar to those of tianeptine the subjects are expected to press the right pedal to get food. In this study the subjects experience a fluoxetine injection similar to that of tianeptine in a certain dose range. In other words, tianeptine and fluoxetine created similar discriminative properties in rats (figure 14).

These results also indicate that tianeptine and fluoxetine may have important similarities in terms of their behavioral mechanisms of action.

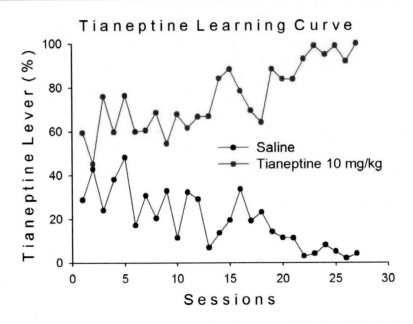

Figure 13. Discrimination of tianeptin (10 mg/kg) from saline. Although at the beginnig of the study rats' ability to discriminate tianeptin from saline was varying between 30-50 % at the end it reached to nearly 100%. Vertical axis of the graph shows percentage pressing of samples on tianeptin arm (n=7; TNP=Tianeptin) (Alici et al, 2006).

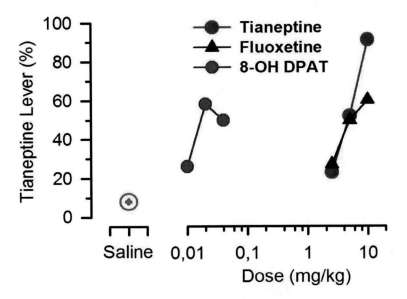

Figure 14. Fluoxetine shows tianeptin like effects on rats trained for tianeptin at a certain dose (n=7-9; TNP=Tianeptin) (Alici et al., 2006).

Another interesting finding of this study is the lack of similar discriminative stimulating properties between tianeptin and venlafaxine, a serotonin and noradrenalin reuptake inhibitor, and caffeine, another stimulating substance that antagonizes adenosine (figure 15).

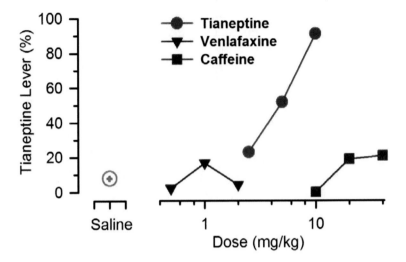

Figure 15. Venlafaxine and caffeine administration to rats trained for tianeptinedoes not show tianeptine like effect (n=7-9; TNP: Tianeptine) (Alici et al., 2006).

These findings show that tianeptine's discriminative properties are not associated with caffeine-like psychostimulation. In addition, there are expected to be differences between the mechanisms of action of tianeptin and another antidepressant, venlafaxine.

Neuroplasticity Hypothesis

A decrease in hippocampal volume in patients with recurrent, refractory depressions or in those having unipolar depression or long-lasting depression, while there is no change in hippocampal volume in young patients with less depressive episodes (Sala et al, 2004), indicates that depression may be associated with structural changes and degeneration in important central regions like the hippocampus as much as with direct changes in the synaptic activities of neurochemicals like monoamines. Starting from these observations, attempts are made to explain the mechanism of depression using changes in neuroplasticity, and the neuroplasticity hypothesis of depression is proposed (Fuchs et al, 2004; Castren, 2005).

This hypothesis explains depression via structural changes in the brain and remodeling in some critical areas like the hippocampus due to these changes rather than the amounts of neurotransmitters released into the synaptic space, their metabolism and their effect on the postsynaptic region via receptors or other ways. This remodeling occurs due to a change in brain neuroplasticity. Besides monoamines like noradrenalin and serotonin, changes in the amounts of several excitatory neurotransmitters like glutamate are also associated with remodeling related functional impairment. Antidepressant treatment primarily reverses this remodeling in addition to stabilizing the impaired monoaminergic balance. During chronic antidepressant treatment a normalized state of neuron structure and synapses is maintained due to the neuroprotective effect (Fuchs et al, 2004). In the following sections of this book the development of depression and the mechanisms of action of antidepressants will be discussed in detail in the context of neuroplasticity.

Chapter 4

Neuroplasticity

What is Neuroplasticity?

Most of the neurons in humans are formed in the late second trimester in prenatal life. Neuronal migration begins in the first weeks of gestation and is nearly finished at term. Indeed, the development of the human brain is more dynamic in the prenatal period and in the early postnatal period than in adult periods. Synapse formation is very rapid from birth to approximately 6 years of age. Beginning from the age of 14 the number of synapses gradually decreases (Stahl, 2000).

This decrease continues throughout life although it slows to a certain level. As the number of synapses decreases the ability of neurons to regenerate and repair themselves continues along with new neuron formation. Formerly, it was thought that besides the decrease in the number of synapses the ability of neurons to regenerate themselves was also lost and no new neurons were formed. Today the opposite has been proved to be the case.

The central nervous system has the ability to adapt both exogenous and endogenous stimuli. Many important central functions are executed with this adaptation, and insufficient adaptation causes the emergence of several diseases. Neuroplasticity can be defined shortly as changes in the brain's neurons and structural and functional changes in synapses formed by these neurons. If the changes are not confined to a single neuron but reach the level of a synapse the adaptive response formed may also be called 'synaptic plasticity'.

Variability of synaptic activity plays a role in the adaptation of the nervous system. The behavioral effects of hormones may be examples of endogenous variations. It has long been known that animal sexual behavior is associated with periodically released hormones and that these hormones exert their effects by changing synaptic activity (Cotman and Nieto-Sampedro, 1984). Adaptation to environmental changes may only be accomplished by learning, and learning requires synaptic plasticity. Learning is the strongest and most important adaptive response of the central nervous system to endogenous and exogenous stimuli. LTP formation in neurons is necessary for learning. LTP formation is an adaptive response associated with neuroplasticity and synaptic plasticity. Although chronic and severe stress causes negative neuroadaptive changes like depression, short term and limited stress is necessary for LTP, which forms the basis for learning. As shown in this discussion, neuroplasticity can cause positive as well as negative changes.

The aplysia is one of the animals most commonly used to examine synaptic mechanisms of learning. This snail rapidly withdraws its gills when a tactile stimulus is applied to its tail or siphon. A decrease in response is observed if the stimulus is repeated. This habituation is explained by a decrease in the efficiency of synapses between sensory and motor neurons. If an electric shock is applied to the tail of the aplysia simultaneously with a tactile stimulus to its siphon a stronger and longer gill withdrawal response is observed with subsequent tactile stimuli. This phenomenon, namely sensitization, is explained by an increase in the efficiency of synapses between sensory and motor neurons (Feldman, 1997).

Some physical changes may appear in the whole neuron or in a part like the dendrite due to neuroplasticity. In addition, new neuron formation, changes in neurons' resistance to negative factors like chronic severe stress and an increase or decrease in synaptic activity may appear. Changes in the central nervous system associated with neuroplastic responses are seen in Table 1. Depending on the strength and length of the stimulus and the properties of primary responding region, one, several or all of these changes may appear. The quality of the resulting neuroplasticity and remodeling due to it also depend on these factors. New neuron formation is called neurogenesis. Neurogenesis is observed most often in the hippocampus and olfactory region. Increases in hippocampal volume and neurogenesis are seen with every mental exercise and chronic stress causes decreases in hippocampal volumes and neurogenesis of hippocampal neurons (Stahl, 2000; Czeh et al, 2001).

Neurotrophic factors are always released in very low concentrations and sometimes they change neurotransmitter-mediated central neurochemical transmission. Some psychotropic drugs may act on central neurotrophic factors besides neurochemical transmission (Carvey, 1998). Some of the important neurotrophic factors known to be present in the central nervous system are seen in Table 2. Neurotrophic factors do not function as neurotransmitters in the central nervous system; primarily they help the development and regeneration of neurons and they contribute to important neuron pathways for structural health and maintaining function. Neurotrophic factors have important roles in the central nervous system for programming and execution of apoptosis. Deficiency of certain neurotrophic factors specific to certain neurons due to endogenous or exogenous reasons triggers a biological cascade resulting in the death of that neuron or group of neurons (Carvey, 1998; Stahl, 2000).

Table 1. Neuroplasticity-induced changes in the brain

Increase or decrease in dendritic branching
Breakage of dendrites
Increase in dendritic length
New synapse formation or disappearance of present synapses
Change in synaptic efficiency of present synapses (Increase or decrease)
Neurogenesis
Apoptosis
Changes in main brain metabolites
Changes in survival of present neurons (increase or decrease)
Increased resistance of neurons to breakage under stress
Changes in stimulus-induced postsynaptic potentials of present neurons
Changes in activities of neurotrophic factors (increase or decrease)

The oldest and most widely known neurotrophic factor is nerve growth factor (NGF), isolated in the fifties by Rita Levi Montalcini. It is the best characterized member of the neurotrophins. NGF gene is located on Chromosome 1 (p21-p22.1 region). NGF has been found in the cortex, the hippocampus, the pituitary gland and the spinal cord. It was shown to promote the survival of primary sensory neurons, and of sympathetic and cholinergic neurons of the basal forebrain (Shoval and Weizman, 2005).

It has been suggested that NGF has a prominent role in the pathophysiology and pharmacotherapy of some neurodegenerative disordes such as Alzheimer type senil dementia (Allen et al., 1991; Backman et al., 1997).

Table 2. Some of the important neurotrophic factors present in the central nervous system

Nerve growth factor (NGF)
Brain-derived neurotrophic factor (BDNF)
Neurotrophin 3 (NT-3)
Neurotrophin 4/5 (NT-4/5)
Neurotrophin-6 (NT-6)
Neurotrophin-7 (NT-7)
Transforming growth factor b3 (TGF-b3)
Basic fibroblast growth factor (bFGF)
Acidic fibroblast growth factor (aFGF)
Glia-derived neurotrophic factor (GDNF)
Ciliary neurotrophic factor (CNTF)
Cholinergic development factor (CDF)
Platelet-derived neurotrophic factor (PDNF)
Insulin-dependent growth factor (IDGF)
Epidermal growth factor (EGF)
Proapoptotic receptors (P75)
Antiapoptotic receptors (TrkA)

Adopted from Carvey, 1998; Stahl, 2000; Sah et al, 2003; Shoval and Weizman, 2005.

Brain-derived neurotrophic factor (BDNF) is a basic dimeric protein. BDNF's gene is located on Chromosome 11, bad p13 (Maisonpierre et al., 1991). This gene has been proposed as a possible source of malfunction in signal transduction from monoamine receptors (Kuipers et al., 2005). BDNF is structurally related to NGF, but it is more widespread in the central nervous system than NGF. Like NGF, BDNF is widespread in the hippocampus (Shoval and Weizman, 2005). Hippocampal damage has been shown to upregulate BDNF level in that region (Ballarin et al., 1991). BDNF has important roles in neurons' survival, maintaining their viability and executing their functions. Normally, BDNF sustains the viability of brain neurons, but the expression of this gene is inhibited under stress. The possibility that BDNF contributes to the action of antidepressant treatment has been supported by behavioral studies of recombinant BDNF and transgenic mouse models. Microinfusion of BDNF into hippocampus produces an antidepressant response in the learned helpness and forced swimming test model of depression (Shirayama et al., 2002; Duman, 2004). The antidepressant effect of BDNF is observed after a single infusion, and is relativelylong-lasting.

Transgenicoverexpression of a dominant negative mutant of the BDNF receptor, trkB, in the hippocampus and other forebrain structures is also reported to block the effect of antidepressant treatment, demonstrating that BDNF signalling is necessary for an antidepressant response (Saarelainen et al., 2003). As more importantly, decreased plasma BDNF levels have been found in depressive patients in recent clinical studies (Aydemir et al., 2006, Kim et al., 2007). Furthermore, decreased levels of BDNF were reversed after antidepressant escitalopram therapy (Aydemir et al., 2006).

Increasing BDNF expression-induced glutamate receptor activation may also be a new target for the treatment of depression. Memantine that modulates glutamate transmission increases BDNF expression. Riluzole, a sodium channel blocker, also increases BDNF expression and neurogenezis in rat hippocampus Marvanova et al., 2001; Katoh-Semba et al., 2002).

Neurotrophin-3 (NT-3)'s gene, located on Chromosome 12 band p13 (Maisone et al., 1991). NT-3 has a role in early neuronal development and that it would be a putative candidate for taking part in the pathophisiology of neurodevelopmental disorders such as schizophrenia (Shoval and Veizman, 2005). It also enhances dopaminergic neuron survival (Gall et al., 1992), indicating a possible role in the pathophysiology of other dopaminergic-related neuropsychiatric disorders such as Parkinson's disease and Tourette's syndrome.

Neurotrophin-4/5 (NT-4/5)'s gene is localized in human chromosome 19 band q 13.3 (Ip et al., 1992). It consists of two identical 130 amino acid subunits sharing 48% sequence identity to NGF and also related to BDNF. It is involved in the promotion of nerve growth and hippocampal cultures synaptic activity (Yin et al., 2001a,b; Schwyzer et al., 2002; Shoval and Weizman, 2005).

Neurotrophin-6 (NT-6) and neurotrophin-7 (NT-7) have been identified only in lower vertebrates. Any relevance of NT-6 and NT-7 to human neurophysiology, neuropathology or possible role in treatment is yet to be elucidated (Shoval and Weizman, 2005).

Neurotrophin receptors are widely expressed in the central nervous system and in the peripheral nervous system, both during brain development in adults. There are two known classes of neurotrophin receptors: The neurotrophin tyrosine kinase receptors (Trk) (high affinity) and the neurotrophin receptor p75^{NTR} (low affinity) (Levin and Barde, 1996; Shoval and Weizman, 2005).

Trks are transmembranal proteins, prosesing and intirinsic tropomyosin related kinase activity. Three different Trks have been found. They are TrkA, TrkB and TrkC. TrkA has the highest affinity for NGF, TrkB has the highest affinity for BDNF and NT-4/5, while TrkC has the highest affinity for NT-3 (Chao et al., 1998; Shoval and Weizman, 2005).

Neurotrophins also bind, with lower affinity, to the p75^{NTR} receptor. Its exact role is not clear, but it has been found to mediate the migration of Schwan cells explants. Interestingly TrkA and p75^{NTR} were shown to collaborate to generate high affinity binding sites for NGF (Chao and Hempstead, 1995). p75^{NTR} seems to act as a co-receptor modulating Trk signalling. Ths functional croostalk between Trk and p75^{NTR} appears to be a key prosesses in the role of neurotropins in the nervous system (Kaplan and Miller, 2000).

Various psychotrop drugs have neuroprotective effects via affecting some neurotrophic factors and elements involved in signal transduction in neuronal membranes. Some of them are listed in Table 3.

Table 3. Neuroprotective effects of drugs

Drugs	Neuroprotection from	Neuropotection suggested to involve
Lithium	Glutamate toxicity β-Amyloid toxicity Oxidative stress MPP+	Bcl2, GSK-3, CREB, BDNF
Valproate	MPP+	Bcl2, GSK-3, BDNF, MAPK
AtypicalNeuroleptics	StressOxidative stress	BDNF, FGF-2, SOD-1
Dopamine Receptor Agonists	Oxidative stress L-DOPA-induced apopitosis	Bcl2, SOD, gluthatione, caspase3
Antidepressants	Stress Glutamate toxicity	cAMP, CREB, BDNF, GDNF
Antibiotics	Stroke Glutamate toxicity	Caspase1, nitric oxide synthase

Adopted from Shamir et al., 2005; Bcl2: B-cell lymphoma, BDNF: Brain-derived neurotrophic factor; cAMP: Adenosine 3', 5'-cyclic monophosphate; CREB: cAMP response element binding protein; FGF-2: Fibroblast growth factor 2; GDNF: Glia-derived neurotrophic factor; GSK-3: Glycogen synthase kinase-3; MAPK: Mitogen-activated protein kinase; SOD: Superoxide dismutase.

Association between Stress and Depression

Publication of the first report and the beginning of the discussion of the detrimental effects of stress took place in the first quarter of the last century. Firstly, it was shown that chronic and heavy stress causes gastric ulceration and hypertrophy of the adrenal gland (Selye, 1976). The detrimental effects of stress on the brain and behavior started to be discussed in the sixties. In the late sixties the suggestion that the hippocampus, a medial temporal structure, is the most sensitive region in the brain regarding binding of glucorticoids to receptors specific for them both in humans and rats formed the basis for the association between stress and psychiatric disorders (McEwen, 1968; McEwen and Weiss, 1970). Glucocorticoids are released in response to stress. Glucocorticoid release is also elevated in major depression and in Cushing's disease (Brown et al, 1999; Starkman et al, 2003).

These findings indicate that conditions that cause stress to living organisms may be associated with depression. Recent studies clearly showed that hippocampal functions are modulated by hormones and neurotransmitters like glutamate, and both glucocorticoid and glutamate levels are increased during conditions that cause stress (McEwen et al, 2002; Moghaddam, 2002; Popoli et al, 2002). Recent studies also suggested that increased glucocorticoid levels and stressful living trigger depressive symptoms (Bayer, 2000; Moghaddam, 2002; Parker et al, 2003).

Depression affects many brain structures. Brain changes with major depression have been reported for the hippocampus amygdale, caudate nucles putamen and frontal cortex, structures that are all extensively interconnected. They comprise a neuroanatomical circuit called the limbic-cortical-striatal-pallidal-thalamic tract.

In view of this, the hippocampal changes have to be seen in a broader context, since it is unlikely that disturbed neurogenezis and structural changes in the hippocampus under the stress will fully explain a disorder as complex as major depression (Fuchs, 2009). It has been suggested that the pathogenesis of depression involves injured hippocampal neurogenezis. In animal models, chronic stress dramatically reduces hippocampal neurogenezis and increases apoptosis in the hippocampal and cortical neurons. It has also been shown that some antidepressants prevented these effects of chronic stress in animals (Czeh et al., 2001; Schmidt and Duman, 2007; Zoladz et al., 2008). On the other hand, stress is known to significantly affect learning and memory processes. These effects are dependent on the type, duration and intensity of the stressor. Emotional arousal may enhance learning and memory through synaptic activity of amygdale-related pathways and this is thougt to be the basis of intense, long term memories of traumatic events and posttraumatic stress disorder (Duman, 2004). Given that the hippocampus is sensitive to stress and glucocorticoids are released during stress, stress-induced hippocampal changes are very important in depression development and as a target of antidepressant drugs. Using these findings as a basis, experimental models based on stress have been formed and both stress-induced changes in elements of neuroplasticity and the effects of antidepressant treatment on these changes have been rigorously examined. Research on this topic is increasing day by day and is growing in importance.

Synaptic Plasticity, Stress and the Effects of Antidepressant

Stress is one of the most important stimuli affecting the central nervous system. The brain has the capacity to adapt to stress-induced changes. Only under chronic stress is the brain's capacity to adapt insufficient at several levels. This insufficiency may cause diseases that originate from the central nervous system (e.g., depression) due to negative remodeling of neuronal quality and neuronal organization. However, the development of important central functions like learning and recovery from diseases (by reversion of remodeling) also requires neuroplasticity. Chronic restrain stress may cause breakage of the dendritic structures in the rat hippocampus as seen in figure 16. In parallel with this, impaired neurogenesis characterized by decreases in hippocampal volume and neurotrophic factors (like BDNF), neuronal atrophy and death may be observed. This may also be interpreted as negative neuroplasticity. This negative neuroplasticity in the brain may be reversed by chronic antidepressant treatment. According to this view, under chronic stress structural defects in the hippocampal CA3 region (neuronal atrophy) and dentate gyrus and a decrease in neurogenesis also occur besides an increase in glucocorticoid levels. This negative neuroplasticity causes depression, and antidepressant treatment ameliorates depression by decreasing neuronal atrophy and increasing neurogenesis (figure 17).

Significant increases occur in dendritic lengths, hippocampal volume, BDNF amount and neurogenesis with antidepressant treatment (Magarinos et al, 1999; Czeh et al, 2001; Duman, 2002; Fuchs et al, 2002; McEwen et al, 2002). Positive effects of antidepressants on neuroplasticity in the rat hippocampus, especially CA3 neurons, after chronic stress are shown in figure 15, 16 and 17.

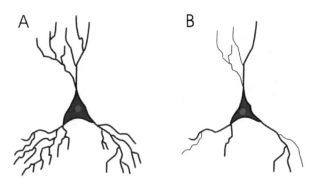

Figure 16. Dendritic changes in rat hippocampal neurons before (A) and after (B) exposure to stress.

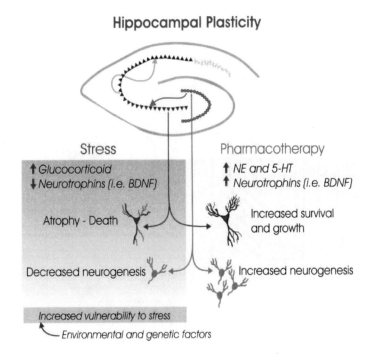

Figure 17. Hippocampal neuroplasticity in depression and effects of the antidepressants.

Breakage of Dendrites Due to Stress and the Effects of Antidepressants

Magarinos et al (1999) observed shortening of dendritic length in pyramidal neurons of the CA3 region of rats exposed to stress caused by restrain stress for three days. Then fluoxetine and tianeptin was applied to rats exposed to similar stress of the same severity and duration. In contrast to the observation that dendritic lengths return to normal in tianeptine administered rats, fluoxetine was not found to be effective. The results of this study indicate that stress-induced remodeling of dendrites may be reversed by an antidepressant, tianeptine. The lack of effect with another depressant, fluoxetine, in this study suggests that the two antidepressants differ with regard to the mechanisms of action of their effects on stress-induced remodeling of dendrites (Figure 18).

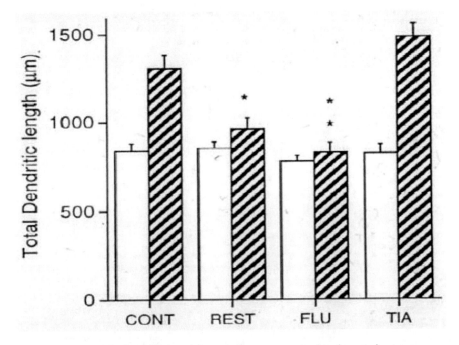

Figure 18. Decrease in dendritic length in rats after exposure to chronic restrain stress (Cont=Control; Rest=Restrain stress; Flu=Fluoxetine; Tia=Tianeptin; *p<0.05 (statistically significant) (Magarinos et al, 1989).

Stress, Hippocampal Volume and the Effects of Antidepressants

Another form of stress-induced neuroplastic remodeling in the central nervous system is volume changes. In studies using magnetic resonance imaging, selective volume decreases were detected in the hippocampus (Sheline, 2000; Sheline et al, 2003; Manji et al, 2003). Ohl et al (2000) showed in a study on three shrews that chronic psychosocial stress and long-term cortisol administration cause important changes in hippocampal volume.

mm³

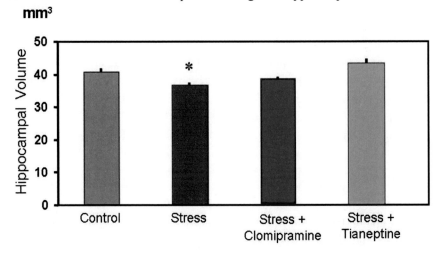

Figure 19. Decrease in rat hippocampal volume due to chronic stress and effect of clomipramine and tianeptin treatment on this (Czeh et al, 2001; van der Hart et al, 2002).

Several subsequent experimental studies also supported the view that chronic exposure to stress causes decreases in hippocampal volume in experimental animals. A more important and interesting result is the reversion to normal of the changes in hippocampal volume due to stress with antidepressant drugs (Figure 19) (Czeh et al, 2001; van der Hart et al, 2002).

The mechanism of stress-induced hippocampal volume decreases has not been clearly identified. However, some probable mechanisms may be discussed. Oversecretion of cortisol may be the first to come to mind. Corticosteroids, with increased release under recurrent stress, may be thought to suppress the hippocampus. However, postmortem studies in the brains of people who used steroids for a long time do not suggest a significant neuronal degeneration or neuropathology. Moreover, very limited apoptosis was observed in the brain following exposure to high levels of corticosteroids. Limited apoptosis is observed in the entorhinal cortex, subiculum, and dentate gyrus. No significant degeneration or other change is detected in the hippocampal CA3 region after high-dose steroid administration (Lucassen et al, 2001a; Muller et al, 2001). These findings are also consistent with studies on other species that found no association between hypercortisolemia and hippocampal neurotoxic effects (Vollman-Hansdorf et al, 1997; Levrenz et al, 1999; Sousa et al, 2000). When we take all these findings into account we conclude that hippocampal volume changes observed in depression cannot be associated with increased corticosteroid release.

Another possible explanation for hippocampal volume changes involves the impairment of neurogenesis under stress. However, hippocampal neurogenesis occurs in a relatively small number of neurons and only at a level that compensates for the neurons that died in the granular layer (Fuchs et al, 2004). If amount and location are taken into account, stress-induced impairment of hippocampal volume will not be expected to occur at a level large enough to be detected by the available methods. However, it is possible that long exposure to stress or impairment in neurogenesis accompanying severe and long-lasting depression may cause this kind of change over time. This hypothesis needs to be supported by thorough experimental and clinical studies. Stress-induced changes in the glial cells of the hippocampal neuron network or dendritic, axonal and synaptic components may also contribute to hippocampal volume loss. In addition, a more mechanistic approach may show that stress-induced changes in the fluid balance between ventricles and brain tissue also cause volume loss. Although studies that suggest ventricular enlargement and loss in several brain tissues in patients with different psychiatric disorders partially support this hypothesis, it would be very speculative to try to explain hippocampal volume loss solely with changes in the fluid balance between the ventricles and brain tissue. As a result, time and further studies are required to explain the causes of hippocampal volume loss in depression or due to stress more clearly.

Stress, Brain Metabolites and the Effects of Antidepressants

Locally applied proton magnetic resonance spectroscopy (MRS) can be used in the research and evaluation of neuropsychiatric disorders. A major advantage of this method is its noninvasiveness (Kato et al, 1998). Proton MRS permits the in vivo measurement of brain metabolites. With this method concentrations of N-acetyl-aspartate (NAA), a neuroaxonal marker of viable and functional capacity of neurons; creatine and phosphocreatine (Cr), an important energy substrate for all cells; compounds including choline (Cho) such as phosphocholine, an important element of cell membrane; and cerebral metabolites such as myo-inositol (ins), an important marker of astrocytes, can also be measured (Birken and Oldendorf, 1989; Urenjak et al, 1993; Brand et al, 1993).

Czeh et al (2001) examined the effects of one week of chronic psychosocial stress on cerebral metabolites such as NAA, Cr, Cho and Ins in tree shrews using proton MRS. They found significant decreases in NAA, Cr and Cho concentrations due to chronic stress. These decreases suggest mainly a decrease and/or functional impairment in neuroaxonal cell density accompanied by a significant impairment in synaptic plasticity. Applying antidepressants together with stress is shown to normalize decreases in NAA, Cr and Cho levels (figure 20).

These observations suggest that cerebral metabolites such as NAA, Cr and Cho may be used for the assessment of stress-induced synaptic plasticity impairment. In addition, these findings support the neuroplasticity hypothesis of depression. Moreover, monitorization of NAA, Cr and Cho levels via MRS appears to indicate the effectiveness of antidepressant therapy.

Czeh et al (2001) observed no significant changes in Ins level either with stress or during antidepressant therapy. Given that Ins is an important marker for astrocytes chronic stress,and depression may be thought to have no significant effect on astrocytes.

Astrocytes, together with oligodendrocytes and microglia, are important elements of the brain's glia. Their proportion in the glia is higher than that of oligodendrocytes and microglia. They form about one third of brain tissue.

Astrocytes play roles in the regulation and execution of many functions very important for synaptic plasticity such as establishing ionic homeostasis in extracellular space, neurotransmitter metabolism, neuronal feeding, providing energy to neurons, regulation of neuronal migration, and secretion of neurotrophic factors. Astrocytes also have an important role in blood brain barrier formation. A new and exciting discovery about astrocytes is their possession of receptors for neurotransmitters and steroid hormones. These receptors do not have many features different from receptors located in neuron membranes, and if they are stimulated with appropriate steroids or neurotransmitters postreceptor biological and electrical events are triggered inside astrocytes. Astrocytes may also coordinate Ca mediated signal transduction (Fuchs et al, 2004).

As Czeh et al (2001) found no significant changes in Ins due to chronic stress it is not possible to determine whether antidepressant treatment is effective at the astrocyte level or not. The resistance of the glia and especially astrocytes to chronic stress should also be kept in mind. Assessment of cerebral Ins levels with more severe stress models other than psychosocial stress or more prolonged psychosocial stress may bring more clarity to this subject.

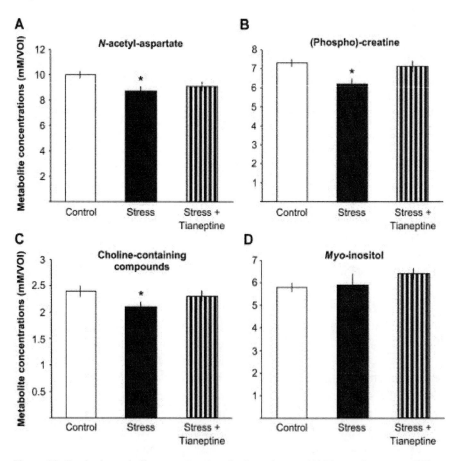

Figure 20. Cerebral metabolite concentrations in three shrews; (A) N-acetyl aspartate; (B) phospho creatine; (C) choline containing compounds and (D) myo-inositol. Control (n=6), stress (n=6) and stress+tianeptin (n=6). Metabolite concentration şs given as mean ±standard deviation (mM/VOI). *p<0.05 differecnce from he control is statistically significant (Czeh et al, 2001).

Stress, Hippocampal Neurogenesis and the Effects of Antidepressants

Increasing evidences have been accumulated during recent years suggesting a role for antidepressant drugs as hippocampal neurogenesis enhancers. The dentate gyrus region of the hippocampus displays an adult neurogenesis characterized by cell death and neogenesis replacing death cells. In this region there is a continuous turnover due to death and regeneration of cells (Biebl et al, 2000; Kuhn et al, 2001). Premature cells produced in the subgranular layer of the hippocampus migrate to the granular layer, where they transform into mature cells. These neurons newly generated in the granular layer have morphologic and physiologic features similar to those of mature neurons previously found in the granular layer (van Praag et al, 2002). Adult hippocampal neurogenesis is shown in many warm-blooded animals and mammals, including humans (Groos, 2000). Interestingly, hippocampal neurogenesis is affected by pharmacological stimulants as well as stimulants from inside and outside (peripheral) the organism (Fuchs and Gould, 2000; Eisch, 2002). For example, stress, as a stimulant both inner and outer or peripheral, may suppress the viability and reproduction of hippocampal granular neurons (Gould et al, 1997; Czeh et al, 2002; Pham et al, 2003; Heine et al, 2004).

Marking with 5-bromo-2'deoxyuridine (BrdU) is used to assess hippocampal neurogenesis. Twenty-four hours after the intraperitoneal application of 100 mg/kg BrdU to rats, staining of healthy dendrites in hippocampal slices with BrdU may easily be seen (figure 21). Decreases in neurotrophic factors and dendritic extensions of neurons or atrophies characterized by dendritic breakage result in decreases in neuron numbers that may be marked by BrdU. This method can be used to show increases or decreases in neurogenesis (Gould et al, 1997; Gould, 1999; Czeh et al, 2001).

In rats chronic stress causes prominent decreases in the number of BrdU stained cells, especially in the hippocampal CA3 region, suggesting a significant decrease in neurogenesis in this region.

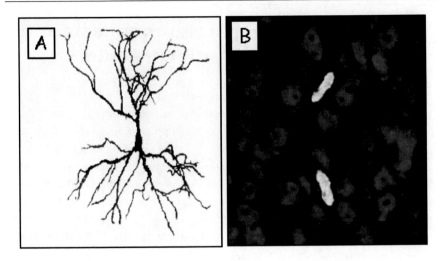

Figure 21. Image of healthy dendrites (A) and a healthy neuron stained with bromodeoxyuridine (B).

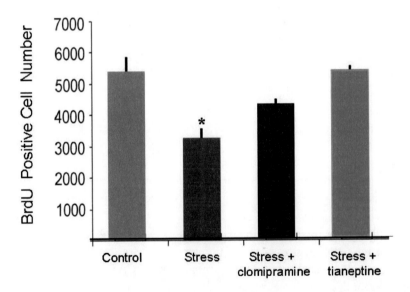

Figure 22. Antidepressant drugs prevent stress induced decrease in neurogenesis in hippocampal CA3 region (BrdU= Bromodeoxyuridine; Czeh et al, 2001; van der Hart et al, 2002).

In 2001, Czeh showed decreased neurogenesis in the hippocampal region due to stress caused by chronic movement restriction can be normalized by an antidepressant, tianeptine in rats (Czeh et al., 2001). In a subsequent study using the same design, van der Hart tested the effects of another antidepressant, clomipramine, and obtained the same results (van der Hart, 2002) (Figure 22). Mostany et al. (2008) also studied in the adult rat hippocampus the effects of chronic treatment with the dual reuptake inhibitor (SNRI) venlafaxine on both cellular proliferation rate and expression of key effectors of several signaling pathways. Increased cell proliferation (BrdU incorporation) in subgranular zone was achieved after chronic treatment with a high dose (40 mg/kg/day) of venlafaxine. However, significant increases in the immunoreactivity of hippocampal beta-catenin in subgranular zone were already detected after administration of a lower dose of the drug (10 mg/kg/day).

These findings clearly show that various antidepressant drugs are able to increase neurogenezis in rat brain.

The results of both studies suggest impairment of the healthy dendrite structure in hippocampal formation due to stress and its amelioration with antidepressant therapy. They also prove that antidepressants can be used effectively to treat stress-induced impairment of neurogenesis. Other authors also suggest that stress-induced impairment plays an important role in the etiology of depression (Jacobs et al, 2000; Eisch, 2002; Kronenberg, 2003).

Many classic treatments of depression, like lithium and electroconvulsive therapy, and many new generation antidepressant drugs have been shown to induce cytogenesis and neurogenesis in the dentate gyrus. It should be noted that improvements in neurogenesis are achieved not with acute but with chronic treatment (Chen et al, 2000; Madsen et al, 2000; Malberg et al, 2000; Scott et al, 2000). Although these studies strongly suggest an important role of hippocampal neurogenesis in depression and antidepressant treatment, we should keep in mind that for now the evidence is restricted to animal studies. The clinical value of this subject will be better understood with large-scale clinical studies.

Stress, Hippocampal Apoptosis and the Effects of Antidepressant

Apoptosis can be defined briefly as cell death. In brain tissue apoptosis is physiologically the reverse of neurogenesis. Normally, apoptosis and neurogenesis work in concert to enable stability. An increase in one may trigger the other and vice versa. Environmental factors such as stress and endogen factors such as increases in free radicals and glucocorticoids not only decrease neurogenesis but also induce apoptosis. At any site in the brain an increase in apoptosis without accompanying neurogenesis or regression of neurogenesis with ongoing apoptosis results in degeneration and functional losses.

Apoptotic cells may be defined and evaluated using immunohistochemical methods. Taking into account that in major depression an increase in apoptosis may also occur along with neurogenesis, whether neuronal apoptosis occurred and whether this apoptosis responded to antidepressant therapy are also examined in animal models. The most important and comprehensive study on this subject was performed recently by Lucassen and study group, who applied chronic psychosocial stress to tree shrews (Lucassen et al, 2004). The tree shrews were put in cages in pairs, one of which was aggressive and dominant and the other passive and recessive. Thus passive and recessive animals were exposed to psychosocial stress in the form of dominant and aggressive ones for seven days. At the end of the study samples exposed to and not exposed to (controls) stress were sacrificed under ethical conditions and apoptotic cell numbers were detected in the temporal cortex and cornu ammonis and dentate gyrus regions of the hippocampus using in situ end labelization (ISEL) under a microscope after staining with diaminobenzidine (Figure 23). The effect of antidepressant treatment on the observed increase in apoptotic cells induced by stress was also examined. Tianeptine was chosen as the antidepressant and the effects of 28-day chronic treatment were evaluated.

The results suggest that 7 days of psychosocial stress caused increased apoptosis in the hippocampal formation of tree shrews. Chronic antidepressant therapy significantly decreased both apoptosis aggravated by stress and apoptosis in normal samples in the temporal cortex and hippocampus. However, tianeptine did not affect apoptosis increasing with stress in normal samples in the cornu ammonis of the hippocampus or the granular layer of the dentate gyrus (figure 24).

These results indicate that apoptosis of neurons in the temporal cortex and subgranular region is more sensitive to chronic tianeptine treatment. On the other hand, antidepressant treatment had positive effects on apoptosis in addition to increasing neurogenesis and correcting dendritic structural defects. Chronic tianeptine therapy also inhibited apoptosis in the cornu ammonis of normal samples but this effect did not reach statistical significance.

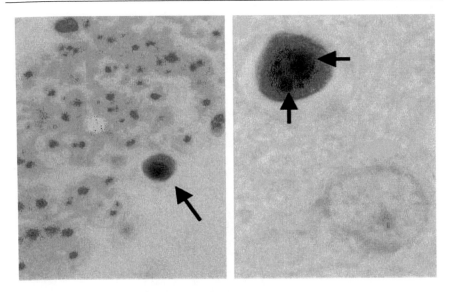

Figure 23. TUNEL-positive apopitotic cells painted with diaminobenzydine in the tree shrew hippocampus (arrows) (adopted from Fuchs et al., 2004).

The insufficient sample size may have had an effect on this. However, one of the most interesting findings of this study was the significant decrease in the total number of marked apoptotic cells in the cornu ammonis compared with controls in contrast to the expected decrease (figure 24).

This decrease may also be the cause of tianeptine's ineffectiveness in the cornu ammonis. The available data did not make it possible for a reasonable explanation to be made for the decrease in apoptosis in the cornu ammonis with stress while it is increasing in other areas. Stress-induced apoptosis may be said to display regional differences. It is clear that more studies are needed for a better understanding of this subject. However, the results of this study definitely show that chronic antidepressant therapy inhibits regionally specific increases in apoptosis.

Another important point that emerged from Lucassen's study is that chronic tianeptine treatment not only inhibited apoptosis induced by stress but also apoptosis in normal samples. This suggests a potential negative effect on organisms' normal apoptosis functions. Inhibition of normal apoptosis may also be associated with increases in certain cells and a carcinogenic effect. Although this approach is highly speculative, antiapoptotic effects should also be considered from this perspective.

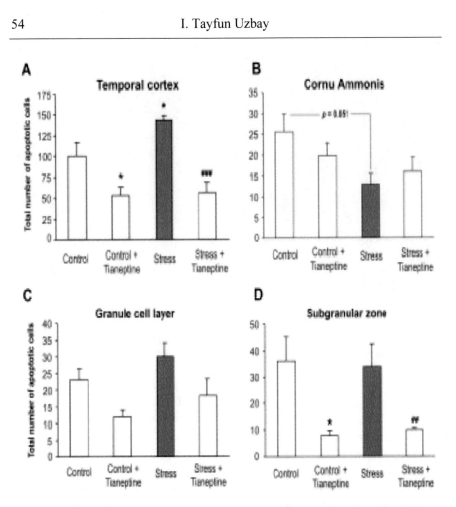

Figure 24. Effects of seven days psychosocial stress on total apoptotic cell numbers in the temporal cortex (A), the cornu ammonis (B), granular layer (C) and subgranular layer (D) of the dentate gyrus. Stress increases apoptosis in the temporal cortex and the dentate gyrus. Chronic tianeptin administration inhibits apoptosis both stress induced and seen in normal controls in the temporal cortex and subgranular dentate gyrus although it is ineffective in other areas (* p<0.05 statistically significant difference from control) (Lucassen et al, 2004).

Stress, Postsynaptic Potential Changes and the Effects of Antidepressant

As previously discussed, learning and memory formation is one of the most effective adaptation mechanisms of organisms against inner and outer stimuli and it is closely associated with long-term potentiation (LTP) emergence, particularly in hippocampal formation. LTP is induction of excitatory postsynaptic plasticity produced by high frequency stimulation of afferent nerve fibers (Diamond et al, 2004). One of the most important observations about the LTP and learning relationship is suppression of LTP and impairment of learning and memory formation by stress longer than a certain time and above a certain severity (Foy et al, 2004).

This observation is confirmed by many subsequent studies (Kim and Diamond, 2002; Diamond et al, 2004). When we consider the importance of learning and memory as a neuroplasticity response, examining the relationship between stress and LTP and the effects of antidepressants on this is a must, regarding the neuroplasticity of depression and the contribution of neuroplasticity to the mechanism of action of antidepressants.

The most comprehensive study examining the effect of stress on LTP and the efficiency of antidepressants on this was conducted by Rocher and his study group (Rocher et al, 2004). In this study rats were kept waiting on a platform elevated 1 meter to induce height anxiety-related acute stress (Figure 25).

In rats waiting on an elevated, narrow platform there was an acute stress reaction characterized by a significant rise in plasma corticosterone levels. As a result, an inhibition in LTP in fibers projecting from the hippocampus to the prefrontal cortex characterized by a decrease in the amplitude of EPSPs was observed. A decrease in EPSP amplitude despite high frequency electrical stimulation indicates disturbance of synaptic plasticity. However, in samples given tianeptine EPSP amplitudes recovered in relation with dose (figure 26).

In this study the maximum tianeptine dose applied did not cause a significant change in high frequency-induced EPSPs in controls not exposed to stress (Figure 27). This suggests that tianeptine's effect is specific to stress-induced changes in neuroplasticity. Rocher et al (2004) evaluated the effects of not only tianeptine but also of fluoxetine. In this part of the study a 10-mg acute dose of either tianeptine or fluoxetine was injected into the nerve pathway between the hippocampus and prefrontal cortex 40 minutes before high frequency electrical stimulation. Changes in EPSPs were evaluated at 30-minute intervals for 2 hours after high frequency stimulation (Figure 27).

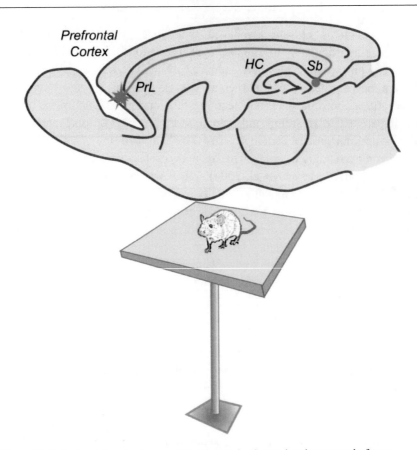

Figure 25. Induction of acute stress reaction in rats in elevated and narrow platforms. Changes in plasma corticosterone levels in rats exposed to stress. The pathways at which excitatory postsynaptic potentials (EPSP) are measured by excitation with high frequency stimulus are seen in the section on upper side of the figure. Assessments are made on glutamatergic fibers that projects directly prelimbic region of prefrontal cortex from CA1 (Sb=Subiculum; PrL= Prelimbic area).

As seen in the figure, both fluoxetine and tianeptine before LTP induction with a high frequency electrical stimulus corrected stress-induced EPSP decreases without causing a change in EPSPs in the examined pathway between the hippocampus and prefrontal cortex. Since neither drug caused a significant change in postsynaptic potentials (PSP) before electrical stimulation their effect is specific to stress-impaired LTP and thus to synaptic plasticity. One of the interesting observations of this study is the longer duration of action of tianeptine on stress-impaired LTP compared with fluoxetin (figure 26). This suggests that there may be therapeutic differences between antidepressants regarding their effects on LTP. Another most important inference from this study is that it forms a basis for explaining stress-induced cognitive impairments with LTP disturbances in neuron networks between the hippocampus and prefrontal cortex.

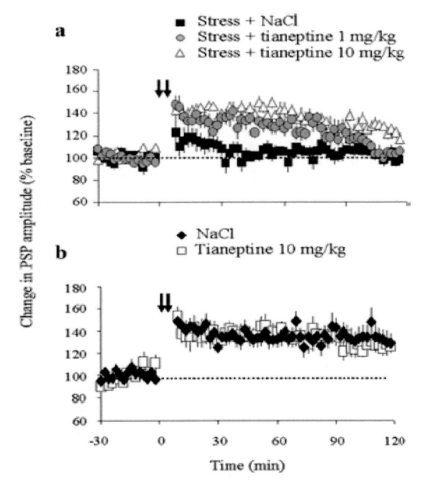

Figure 26. Effects of the antidepressants over stress induced impairment of EPSP amplitudes in fibers that Project from hippocampus to prefrontal cortex. (a) = rats exposed to stress (b) rats not exposed to stress (Rocher et al., 2004).

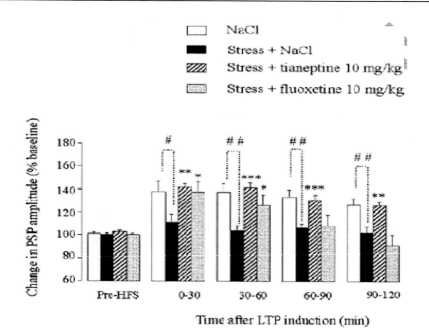

Figure 27. Stress induced changes in EPSP amplitudes due to high frequency electrical stimulus and effects of the antidepressants (Rocher et al, 2004).

Although hippocampal LTP formation is very important for learning and memory, LTP formation is not restricted to the hippocampal formation. Many studies have clearly shown that LTP is formed in many nuclei of the hippocampus (Maren and Fanselow, 1995; Chapman et al, 2003; Yaniv et al, 2003a). Nevertheless, in the amygdala, in contrast to the hippocampus and prefrontal cortex, there is an increase in synaptic transmission and PSP amplitudes of formed EPSPs related to emotional stimuli (Rogan et al, 1997; Blair et al, 2001). A recent experimental study also found that in rats exposed to stress due to staying in an unfamiliar environment despite the decrease in LTP magnitudes in the amygdala low threshold LTP formation was blocked in the hippocampus (Yaniv et al, 2003b). Given that anxiety and fear emerge in conditions at which the amygdala is stimulated, an increase in LTPs in the amygdala with inhibition in the hippocampus and prefrontal cortex may be explained as necessary for survival under stress.

Some preliminary behavioral and electrophysiological studies interestingly indicate that treatment with antidepressants like tianeptine is ineffective on stress-induced LTP changes in amygdala. For example, Burghardt et al. (2004) has shown that fear conditioning, a strong form of emotional learning, is not affected by acute tianeptine administration. Vouimba et al (2003) also showed that a stress-related amygdaloid LTP increase that may be regarded as a reflection of fear conditioning is not changed by tianeptine treatment. According to these data the effects of tianeptine on stress-related LTP change may be thought to be restricted to the hippocampus and prefrontal cortex without affecting the amygdaloid complex. Nevertheless, the effects of other antidepressants on the LTP increases observed under stress should also be examined and taken into account during evaluation.

Some clinical studies indicate that tianeptine effectively treats somatic anxiety symptoms accompanying depression and may have anxiolytic effects (Defrance et al, 1988; Guelfi et al, 1989; Wilde and Benfield, 1995). In this case, the ineffectiveness of tianeptine on increases in LTP induced due to fear and stress may seem controversial. However, measured PSP increases in the amygdala due to fear and stress may be associated with normal anxiety rather than being pathologic. Examining LTP changes in the amygdala and the effects of tianeptine on this in models measuring pathologic anxiety will help us to understand this subject better. However, although some studies indicate that tianeptine has an anxiolytic effect, this study assessed tianeptine's effects on somatic anxiety accompanying major depression rather than its effects solely on anxiety. Controversial results were also obtained in studies conducted on experimental animals with models of solely different types of anxiety (Zethof et al, 1995; Cutler et al, 1997). Effects of tianeptin and other antidepressants on amygdala neuroplasticity should be assessed with further and more detailed studies.

Contribution of Glutamate in Stress Induced Neuroplasticity and the Effects of Antidepressants on Glutamatergic System

Chronic stress not only triggers glucocorticoid release. Recent studies have clearly shown that excitatory amino acidergic system is also stimulated under stress and increases in glucocorticoid release occur in many brain regions especially in hippocampus (Lowy et al, 1993; 1995; Maghaddam et al, 1994). N-methyl-D-aspartate receptors are abundant in the central nervous system and they are among the most important receptors mediating the excitatory effects of glutamate. NMDA receptor antagonists have been shown to increase neurogenesis in dentate gyrus of hippocampus (Cameron et al, 1995) and prevent dendritic remodelling assumed to appear due to stress induced increase in glucocorticoid release (Magarinos et al, 1999; McEwen 1999b). These observations indicate that glutamatergic system may have a key role in the regulation of synaptic plasticity and antidepressants may affect not only monoamines but also other neurotransmitters like glutamate.

Excitatory neuotransmitters like glutamate suppress neurogenesis in dentate gyrus of hippocampus and have a key role breakage of stress induced breakage in hippocampal dendrites. Regulation of the extracellular glutamate levels may be a potential cause of remodelling because of the dendritic disruption and breakage of CA3 region hippocampal neurons induced by chronic stress. Regulation and distribution of glia glutamate transporter (GLT-1) and its isoforms may give an idea about glutamate activity as well as structural disruptions of dendrite and suppression of neurogenesis. A detailed study testing this hypothesis was conducted recently by Reagan and his study group (Reagan et al, 2004). In this study regulation and distribution of glia GLT-1 and one of its isoforms GLT-1b in rat hippocampus that are exposed to chronic restrain stress for 21 days through the restriction of their movements 6 hours a day. In this study, effects of an antidepressant, tianeptin, over chronic stress induced changes in the expression of GLT-1 and GLT-1b is also examined to answer the question whether antidepressants affect the glutamate mediated changes in synaptic plasticity after stress.

Tianeptine was given to the treatment groups (together with stress) by intraperitoneal route at a dosage of 10 mg/kg chronically for 21 days.

Stress application based on chronic movement restriction (restrain stress) results in a significant increase in GLT-1 mRNA levels and protein expression in the hippocampal CA3 region and dentate gyrus of the rat. An important aspect of this study is the assessment of stress-induced changes at different sites and in some detail in the cornu ammonis and dentate gyrus. Indeed, significant increases in GLT-1 mRNA levels and protein expression appeared only in the CA3 region of the cornu ammonis and molecular layer of the dentate gyrus. When the effects of stress in the CA3 region are evaluated in detail, stress-induced increases are seen to be limited to the stratum oriens and stratum radium. No stress-induced change occurred for GLT-1 in the CA3 region of the stratum pyramidalis. Likewise, no stress-induced change was detected in the granular layer of the dentate gyrus or hilus (Figure 28 A and B). These observations suggest that several regions such as CA3 of the hippocampal formation and the molecular layer of the dentate gyrus are more sensitive to chronic stress induced by movement restriction and to changes in glutamate activity due to this. Whether any change in unaffected regions may be seen by using other stress models or by using the same model for longer may only be clear after further studies.

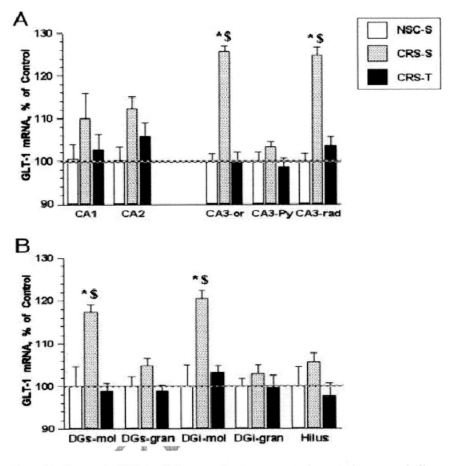

Figure 28. Changes in GLT-1 mRNA expression in rats exposed to restrain stress and effect of tianeptin tretment. (A) Cornu ammonis region; or = stratum oriens, py = stratum pyramidale, rad = stratum radiatum. (B) Dentate gyrus, mol= molecular layer, gran= granular layer, s= superior, i= inferior. NSC-S= non-stress + saline control; CRS-S= chronic stress + tianeotin. * p<0.05 statistically significant from chronic stress + tianeptin (Reagan et al, 2004).

The most important finding of this study is that stress-induced glutamate activity increases can be suppressed by antidepressant treatment (Figure 28 A and B). Tianeptine treatment did not change the GLT-1 mRNA levels or protein expression in hippocampal layers not affected by stress. This finding is important because it shows that antidepressant drugs ameliorate the neuroplastic changes induced by glutamate. It follows from this that antidepressants can affect not only monoamines like noradrenalin and serotonin but also excitatory neurotransmitters like glutamate.

In this study, stress induced by chronic movement restriction did not cause any significant change in GLT-1b (an isoform of GLT-1) mRNA levels in any region of the hippocampus. Moreover, no significant effect of chronic tianeptine (10 mg/kg, ip) treatment was observed (Figure 29). These findings indicate that changes induced by glutamate transporters in the hippocampal formation and tianeptine effects are only limited to GLT-1, and isoforms like GLT-1b are not affected by stress or tianeptine.

Thus, stress causes glutamatergic activity to increase, particularly with GLT-1 increases. This can be prevented by tianeptine and this effect occurs in the hippocampal formation, especially in the CA3 region and dentate gyrus. In addition, it is seen that GLT-1 plays an important role in the effect of tianeptine on glutamatergic regulation.

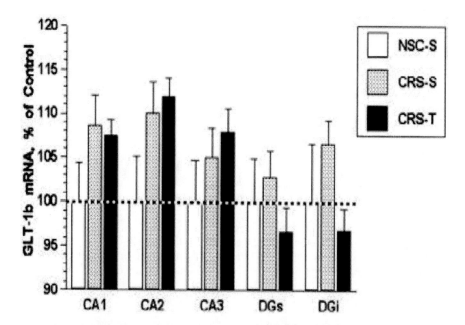

Figure 29. GLT-1b mRNA expression changes in rats exposed to restrain stress and effects of the antidepressants. No significant change is observed in he levels of hippocampal GLT1-b mRNA levels of rats exposed to stress. (CRS-S = Chronic stress + saline; CRS-T = Chronic stress + tianeptin; NSC-S = non stress + saline) (Reagan et al, 2004).

Modulation of glutamatergic transmission by tianeptine is confirmed by the results of electrophysiological studies that investigated the effects of stress-induced changes in the glutamatergic synapses. For example, Kole et al. (2002) showed that tianeptine normalizes NMDA currents augmented by stress in the CA3 region of the hippocampal formation in rats subjected to chronic stress.

Nitric oxide (NO) may also make a modulatory contribution to the effects of antidepressants through glutamate. NO is a labile, free radical gas with a very short half-life (6-10 sec) that has important biological activity both in the periphery and in the central nervous system. It is synthesized by a reaction that uses L-arginine as a precursor and is catalyzed by NO synthase (Snyder and Bredt, 1992). There are three different isoforms of NOS: endothelial (eNOS), inducible (iNOS) and neuronal (nNOS) (Moncada et al., 1997). It is shown that NOS activity is found in many brain regions, including the hippocampus (Forsterman et al., 1990). In addition, based on data showing that NO can be a new and unusual neurotransmitter, the existence of a central L-arginine-NO pathway is suggested (Moncada and Higgs, 1993). Results of several clinical and experimental studies indicate that NO may play a role in other neuropsychiatric diseases like the physical component of alcohol and substance addiction (Uzbay and Oglesby, 2001), schizophrenia (Zoroglu et al., 2002; Yanik et al., 2003), bipolar affective disorders (Savas et al., 2002) and obsessive compulsive disorder (Zoroglu et al., 2003).

It is proposed that in the central nervous system NO interacts with the glutamatergic system and second messenger cGMP contributing to the emergence of excitatory responses like alcohol deprivation syndrome (Uzbay and Oglesby, 2001). According to this view, stimulation of excitatory amino acid receptors, especially NMDA receptors with glutamate, causes Ca^{2+} /calmoduline mediated activation of NOS by increasing the entrance of Ca^{2+} into the cell at the postsynaptic neuronal membrane. Activation of NOS also causes NO synthesis and increases NO production. NO synthesized and released at the postsynaptic neuron diffuses to the presynaptic neuron retrogradely and provokes the glutamate release at the presynaptic terminal by stimulating guanilate cyclase (GC) (Garthwaite et al., 1989; Garthwaite, 1991; Uzbay and Oglesby, 2001) (Figure 30).

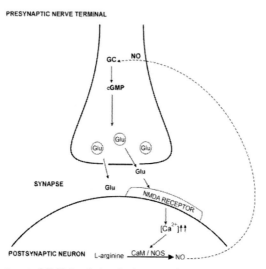

Figure 30. NO- Glutamate-NMDA relation in the central nervous system (Uzbay and Oglesby, 2001).

Increases in striatal L-sitrulline levels in the rat brain (Gören et al., 2001) during alcohol deprivation and significant increases in cGMP levels especially in the hippocampus and striatum during both chronic alcohol intake and alcohol deprivation (Uzbay et al., 2004) are findings that support the contribution of NO to the excitatory symptoms during alcohol deprivation syndrome. Wegener et al. (2003) showed that antidepressants like fluoxetine and tianeptine inhibit NOS, a NO synthesizing enzyme in the central nervous system, and NO activity, especially in the hippocampus. NOS-inhibiting effects of antidepressants in the hippocampus may indirectly augment their inhibitory effect on glutamate activity. Given that NO is a free radical and that excessive NO facilitates cell degeneration, it is expected that the NO-activity-decreasing effects of antidepressants may help to protect neurons. It is known that antidepressants like tianeptine exert their neuroprotective effects by also blocking the increase in lactate dehydrogenase activity induced by hypoxia (Plaisant et al., 2003).

All these observations indicate that antidepressant drugs have some beneficial effects on disorders associated with depression and/or neuronal disorders that cause depression inhibition of the glutamatergic system directly or indirectly. Positive effects on free radicals can also contribute to the neuroprotective effects. Examining the interaction of antidepressants with glutamate and NO will also be of great assistance in the development of more effective psychotropic drugs.

Stress, Neurotrophic Factors and the Effects of Antidepressants

During chronic stress formation and corticosterone administration, an increase in glucocorticoid release is observed, especially in the CA1 and CA3 regions of the hippocampal formation of the brain, while concentrations of important neurotrophic factors like BDNF decrease. These decreases are characterized by a reduction of BDNF mRNA expression (Scaccionoce et al., 2003). A decrease in neurotrophic factor releasing reduces the resistance of neurons to stress. Besides neuronal atrophies due to breakage of dendrites, the balance between neurogenesis and apoptosis is also impaired. As a result, impairment of synaptic plasticity and synaptic transmission is seen (Fossati et al., 2004) (Figure 17). The cause of the BDNF level decrease under stress is suppression of BDNF gene promoter transcription through corticosteroid receptor stimulation (Schaaf et. al., 2000). Dysfunction of cAMP response element (CRE) binding protein (CREB) may also contribute to BDNF deficiency (Dowlatshahi et al., 1998). Goggi et al. (2002) showed that BDNF acutely affects both the electrophysiological aspect of LTP-induced synaptic plasticity and neurochemical aspects through release of neurotransmitters like serotonin and glutamate. Deficiency of BDNF has an important role in the pathology of many affective disorders including depression and schizophrenia (Angellucci et al., 2004). These findings indicate that BDNF is a very important neurotrophic factor both in the development of depression and in antidepressant treatment.

CREB can be activated in vitro by cAMP-protein kinase A (PKA) pathway through the stimulation of 5-HT receptors (Duman et al., 1998) and noradrenergic receptors (Roseboom and Klein, 1995). CREB activity can also be directly induced by Ca^{2+} dependent protein kinases stimulated by adrenergic receptors and serotonergic 5-HT$_2$ receptors (Duman, 1998). CREB activation and subsequent increases in BDNF gene expression have an important role in the antidepressant mechanism of action. Other studies also show that the cAMP/CREB/BDNF system is stimulated and activated by several antidepressants and during electroconvulsive therapy (Nibuya et al., 1995, 1996).

Treatment with antidepressant drugs increases the levels of monoaminergic neurotransmitters like serotonin and noradrenaline at synapses. The neurotransmitters released into the synaptic space activate the signal transduction system between cells by binding to specific receptors.

BDNF and CREB are essential elements of this signal transduction system. Chronic treatment with antidepressants affects several proteins linked to neuroplasticity, particularly BDNF. This statement leads eventually to their therapeutic effects. It is possible that also for putative early therapeutic onset, antidepressants may act by promoting cellular adaptations linked to neuroplasticity (Tardito et al., 2009; Alboni et al., 2010). In an experimental study, it has been shown that antidepressants such as fluoxetine, a selective serotonin reuptake inhibitor, and desipramine, a selective noradrenaline reuptake inhibitor, increased CRE-binding activity in rat frontal cortex when they were administered for 21 consecutive days. Fluoxetine also increased the CRE-binding activity in hippocampus (Frechilla et al., 1998). In a following study, Morinobu et al. (2000) observed that single administration of paroxetine, an SSRI, significantly induced the phosphorylation of CREB in the rat frontal cortex and hippocampus in a time-dependent manner. This data imply that intracellular signal transduction may be involved in the therapetic effect of paroxetine.

Thome et al. (2000) also performed an experimental study with rats and showed that CRE mediated gene expression and CREB phosphorylation increased in various regions of the brain under chronic treatment of desypramine, fluoxetine and tranylcypromin (a monoamine oxidase enzyme inhibitor). Among the three different antidepressants used in this study, fluoxetine is found to be most effective in terms of its influence on CREB phosphorylation. Nevertheless, it is interesting that fluoxetine is ineffective on both CRE-mediated gene expression and CREB phosphorylation in the CA3 region of the hippocampal formation. This may be because this layer of hippocampus does not contribute to the effects of fluoxetine emerging through CRE. Interestingly, fluoxetine, a protype agent of SSRIs, was found to be effective on functional deficits after hypoxic ischemia brain injury in rat pups (Chang et al., 2006). In this study, it has been shown that chronic treatment of fluoxetine could upregulate CREB activation in the hippocampus. The authors also examined whether fluoxetine administration before hypoxic ischemia may protect against neonatal hypoxic ischemia brain injury through CREB-mediated mechanisms. They found that low-dose fluoxetine pretreatment in a neonatal hypoxic ischemia brain injury model significantly reduced functional deficits at adulthood. The neuroprotective mechanisms were associated with increased CREB phosphorylation and increased brain-derived neurotrophic factor and synapsin I mRNA expression in the hippocampus. Neurogenesis also increased because of greater precursor cell survival in the hippocampal dentate gyrus (Figure 31 and 32) (Chang et al., 2006).

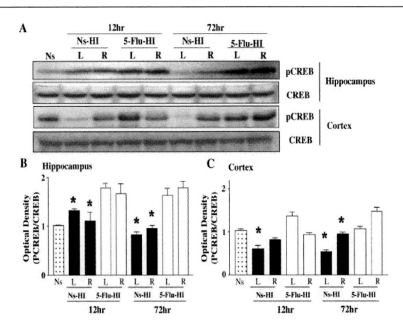

Figure 31. Fluoxetine pretreatment increased CREB phosphorylation (pCREB) in the hippocampus and cortex after hypoxic–ischemia (HI). (A–C) Representative Western blots and the corresponding densitometry of pCREB/CREB ratio showed that the 5-mg/kg-fluoxetine-pretreated (5-Flu-HI) group had significantly higher pCREB levels in the ipsilateral hippocampus 12 h and 72 h after HI than did the normal-saline-pretreated (Ns-HI) group at the respective time point (*both $p < 0.05$). The 5-Flu-HI group also had significantly higher pCREB levels in the ipsilateral cortex 72 h after HI than did the Ns-HI group (*$p < 0.05$). Compared with the Ns-HI group, the 5-Flu-HI group had significantly higher pCREB levels in the contralateral hippocampus and cortex 12 h and 72 h after HI (*all $p < 0.05$). Total CREB was unchanged between the two HI groups. Data are from $n = 5$ experiments in each group. L: left hemisphere, R: right hemisphere, Ns: normal saline controls (from Chang et al., 2006).

These observations imply that functional deficits after hypoxic ischemia in the developing brain can be reduced by antidepressant agents that enhance neural plasticity and neurogenesis through CREB activation.

Tryptophan hydroxylase (TPH) is the rate limiting enzyme in the serotonergic pathway and regulates serotonin levels in mammals. Because seotonin is an important neurotransmitter in depression, investigation of changes in TPH protein expression before and after stress and under the antidepressant treatments could be important. Abumaria et al. (2007) observed that expression of TPH protein upregulated by the stress and normalized by citalopram, an antidepressant in the dorsal raphe nucleus of the rats. In this study, citalopram had no effect on serotonin transporter mRNA but reduced serotonin-1A autoreceptor mRNA in stressed animals. It prevented the stress-induced upregulation of mRNA for CREB binding protein, synaptic vesicle glycoprotein 2b and the glial N-myc downstream-regulated gene 2, but increased mRNA for neuron-specific enolase (NSE) in both stressed and unstressed animals having no effect on stress-induced upregulation of NSE protein. These findings demonstrate that in the dorsal raphe nucleus of chronically stressed rats, citalopram normalizes TPH expression and blocks stress effects on distinct genes related to neurotransmitter release and neuroplasticity.

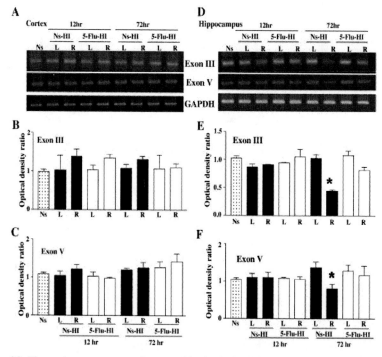

Figure 32. Fluoxetine pretreatment increased brain-derived neurotrophic factor (BDNF) transcription in the hippocampus after hypoxic–ischemia (HI). The levels of both BDNF exon III and exon V mRNA in the cortex were comparable between the normal-saline-pretreated (Ns-HI) and 5-mg/kg-fluoxetine-pretreated (5-Flu-HI) groups (A–C). In contrast, compared with the Ns-HI group, the 5-Flu-HI group had significantly higher expressions of BDNF exon III and exon V mRNA in the ipsilateral hippocampus 72 h after HI (both *$p < 0.05$) (D–F). Data are from $n = 4$–6 experiments in each group. The PCR products of BDNF were normalized to corresponding GAPDH products in each sample. L: left hemisphere, R: right hemisphere, Ns: normal saline controls (from Chang et al., 2006).

As mentioned before, chronic restraint stress affects hippocampal and amygdalar synaptic plasticity as determined by electrophysiological, morphological and behavioral measures, changes that are inhibited by some antidepressants. Reagan et al., (2007) investigated BDNF expression in rat amygdala after chronic restrain stress and tianetine treatment. They observed that, BDNF mRNA expression was not modulated in chronic restraint stress rats given saline in spite of increased pCREB levels. Conversely, BDNF mRNA levels were increased in the amygdala of chronic restraint stress/tianeptine rats in the absence of changes in pCREB levels when compared to non-stressed controls. Amygdalar BDNF protein increased while pCREB levels decreased in tianeptine-treated rats irrespective of stress conditions (figure 33 and 34). Collectively, these findings demonstrate that tianeptine concomitantly decreases pCREB while increasing BDNF expression in the rat amygdala, increases in neurotrophic factor expression that may participate in the enhancement of amygdalar synaptic plasticity mediated by tianeptine, an antidepressant agent. Escitalopram, known to be already effective in preclinical models of depression after 7 days, allowed us to investigate whether two effective treatment regimens (7 and 21 days) may contribute to synaptic plasticity by acting on BDNF signalling. Seven days of treatment with escitalopram activated intracellular pathways linked to BDNF and increased the levels of Pro-BDNF in the rat prefrontal cortex.

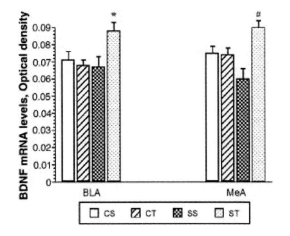

Figure 33. Autoradiographic image analysis of BDNF mRNA expression in the basolateral nucleus of the amygdala and medial nucleus of the amygdala of rats subjected to chronic restraint stress and tianeptine treatment. Statistical analysis revealed that tianeptine treatment increased BDNF mRNA expression in rats subjected to chronic restraint stress; there was no effect due to chronic restraint stress alone. $* = P < 0.05$ compared to non-stressed controls given saline (CS); $\# = P < 0.05$ compared to rats subjected to chronic stress and given saline (SS) (from Reagan et al., 2007).

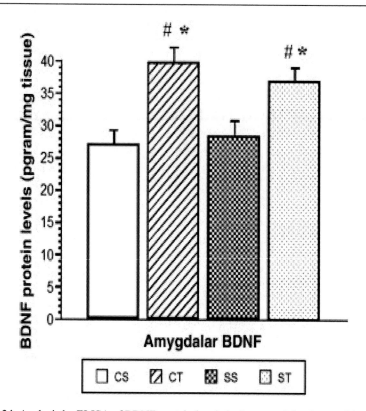

Figure 34. Analysis by ELISA of BDNF protein levels in the amygdala of rats subjected to chronic restraint stress in the presence and absence of tianeptine administration. Statistical analysis revealed that tianeptine treatment increased BDNF protein levels in rats subjected to chronic restraint stress and in non-stressed control rats. $* = P < 0.05$ compared to CS; # $= P < 0.05$ compared to SS (from Reagan et al., 2007).

Furthermore, 21 days of treatment with escitalopram decreased CREB/BDNF signalling while increasing p38 levels in the rat hippocampus (Alboni et al., 2010) (Figure 35 and 36). Even if further experiments with different antidepressant strategies will be needed, this information suggest that escitalopram efficacy may be mediated by early and late effects on synaptic plasticity in selective brain areas. Thus, antidepressants may have different effects on neurohumoral signalling systems in a time-dependent manner.

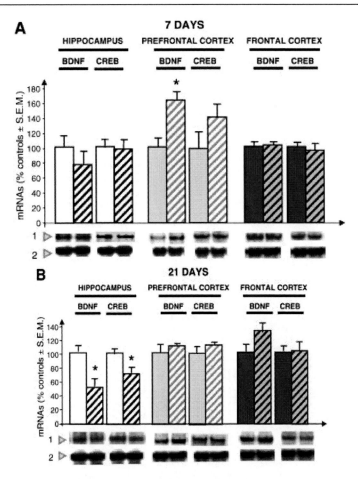

Figure 35. Effect of a subchronic (A-7 days) or a chronic (B-21 days) treatment with escitalopram (10 mg/kg) on the mRNA levels of BDNF and CREB in rat hippocampus, prefrontal cortex and frontal cortex. A) BDNF mRNA was significantly induced in prefrontal cortex of escitalopram-treated rats with respect to saline-treated ones. B) Following a 21 day treatment with escitalopram the mRNA levels of BDNF and CREB were significantly decreased with respect to the group treated with saline in hippocampus. Animals were treated for 7 or 21 days with either escitalopram (10 mg/kg) or saline (1 ml/kg). Rats were sacrificed 18 h after the last injection. The arrow shows representative autoradiographies of an RNase protection assay of target genes (1: BDNF and CREB or 2: internal standard cyclophilin); 15 µg of total RNA was used in each lane. The results, normalized for cyclophilin, were expressed as % of saline-treated animals. Each column represents mean ± S.E.M.; *P < 0.05 with respect to saline group (t-test) (from Alboni et al., 2010).

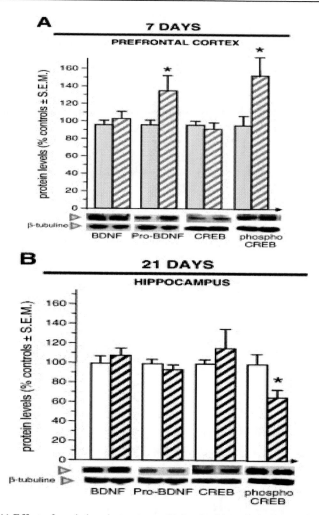

Figure 36. (A) Effect of a subchronic treatment (7 days) with escitalopram on BDNF and CREB protein levels in rat prefrontal cortex. Seven-day exposure to escitalopram significantly increased phospho-CREB and Pro-BDNF levels in prefrontal cortex with respect to animals injected intraperitoneally with saline for a week. (B) Effect of a chronic treatment (21 days) with escitalopram on BDNF and CREB protein levels in rat hippocampus. In the hippocampus of rats treated for 21 days with escitalopram phospho-CREB levels were significantly decreased with respect to the saline group. *Animals were treated for 7 or 21 days with either escitalopram (10 mg/kg) or saline (1 ml/kg). Rats were sacrificed 18 h after the last injection. Total levels of BDNF mature form and Pro-BDNF, CREB and phospho-CREB (p-CREB) in the nuclear enriched fraction were evaluated by western blotting. Arrows show representative immunoblots. CREB, phospho-CREB, BDNF and Pro-BDNF normalized for β-tubuline, were expressed as % of saline-treated animals. Each column represents mean ± S.E.M.; *P < 0.05 with respect to saline group (t-test)* (from Alboni et al., 2010).

Stress, Hippocampal Gene Expression and the Effects of Antidepressants

Using complementary DNA (cDNA) subtractive libraries from cortisol-treated tree shrews, it has been recently identified four genes differentially expressed in the hippocampus of male tree shrews subjected to chronic psychosocial stress. These genes encode the nerve growth factor (NGF), the membrane glycoprotein 6a (M6a), the guanine nucleotide binding protein (G protein) alpha q polypeptide (GNAQ), and a CDC-like kinase 1 (CLK-1). Downregulation of M6a, GNAQ, and CLK-1 messenger RNA (mRNA) expression could be reversed by clomipramine treatment (Alfonso et al 2004). Interestingly, these four genes have been previously related to neurogenesis, neuronal differentiation, and/or neurite outgrowth (Heasley et al 1996, McAllister et al 1999, Mukobata et al 2002 and Myers et al 1994).

In a recent study, Alfonso et al. (2006) evaluated whether these alterations in gene expression are conserved in a different stress animal model. They measured NGF, M6a, GNAQ, and CLK-1 expression levels in the hippocampus of male and female mice from BALB/c and C56BL/6 strains subjected to repeated restraint stress for 3 weeks. In this study, the authors also determined expression levels for other neuronal and synaptic plasticity-related genes such as BDNF, CREB, synaptic associated protein synapsin I, protein kinase C alpha (PKC-α), neural cell adhesion molecule 140 (NCAM-140), and growth associated protein 43 (GAP-43). Finally, to study whether antidepressant treatment can reverse the changes in gene expression observed after exposure to repeated stress, they also subjected animals to chronic restraint stress and daily tianeptine administration, an atypical antidepressant. The results of the study indicated that Chronically stressed mice displayed a reduction in transcript levels for NGF, M6a, GNAQ, and CLK-1. In addition, other genes implicated in neuronal plasticity, such as BDNF, CREB, PKC, NCAM, and synapsin I were downregulated in stressed mice. Tianeptine treatment reversed the stress effects for the genes analyzed. Alterations in gene expression were dependent on the duration of the stress treatment and, in some cases, were only observed in male mice (Figure 37 and 38).

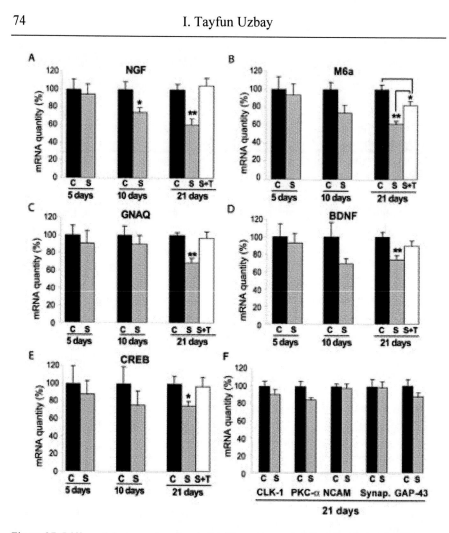

Figure 37. Differential gene expression in the hippocampus is induced only by chronic stress and is reversed by tianeptine treatment. Female BALB/c mice were either untreated control subjects ("C," black bars), subjected to 5, 10, or 21 days of restraint stress ("S," gray bars), or treated with tianeptine concomitantly to the stress procedure ("S+T," white bars). Messenger RNA samples from the hippocampal formation were used for quantification of NGF (A), M6a (B), GNAQ (C), BDNF (D), CREB (E), CLK-1, PKC-α, NCAM-140, synapsin I, and GAP-43 (F) expression levels using real time RT-PCR. Values for each individual were normalized with the reference gene cyclophilin. *p < .05, **p < .01. S+T group value for M6a expression levels is statistically different to both C and S group values. NGF, nerve growth factor; M6a, membrane glycoprotein 6a; GNAQ, guanine nucleotide binding protein (G protein) alpha q polypeptide (Alfonso et al., 2006).

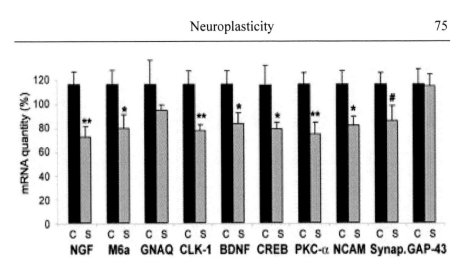

Figure 38. Regulation of gene expression in the hippocampus of chronically stressed male BALB/c mice. Male BALB/c mice were subjected to 21 days of restraint stress ("S," gray bars) or left undisturbed (control subjects: "C," black bars). Messenger RNA samples from the hippocampal formation were used for quantification of NGF, M6a, GNAQ, BDNF, CREB, CLK-1, PKC-α, NCAM-140, synapsin I, and GAP-43 cDNA amounts using real time RT-PCR. Values for each individual were normalized with the reference gene cyclophilin. Plotted data shows mean group values +SEM expressed as a percentage of the respective control group (Alfonso et al., 2006).

Conclusion

Despite acute regulation of monoaminergic neurotransmission, resulting in a significant increase of synaptic monoamine concentrations, most antidepressants still require several weeks before clinical effects occur. This delayed therapeutic action may results from either the indirect regulation of other neuronal signal transduction systems or the regulation of gene transcription. An "initial and adaptation" model has recently been proposed to describe the drug-induced changes of neuronal plasticity associated with the long-term actions of antidepressants in the brain (Hyman and Nestler, 1996; Kuipers et al., 2005).

In the light of the data discussed so far, it is seen that changes in synaptic plasticity that occur in the brain under stress play an important role in the development of neuropsychiatric disorders like depression. The neuroplasticity hypothesis of depression appears to explain depression more accurately than does the monoamine hypothesis. Recently, it was shown that antidepressants like tianeptine that have significant effects on neuroplasticity also have other useful effects such as being anticonvulsants associated with the excitatory amino acidergic system in experimental animals (Ceyhan et al., 2005). This observation highlights the reality that the field of neuroplasticity is widening to include other psychiatric and neurological disorders. It may be expected that drugs that have an effect on neuroplasticity treat not only depression but also other diseases related to the central nervous system and having a neurodegenerative course. This can provide a more effective treatment with fewer drugs for patients who have depression and other diseases with a central origin. Therefore, it will be inevitable to reshape the strategies of psychotropic drug development to concentrate on the development of molecules that affect neuroplasticity to include these mechanisms rather than drugs that modulate the interaction between neurotransmitter release, reuptake and receptor systems (Uzbay, 2008).

An important point concerning neuroplasticity and the effects of psychotropic drugs that should not be neglected is that available studies were conducted on experimental animals and are limited in number. Moreover, most of the studies evaluate the effects of tianeptine only. Although there are some data about fluoxetine and tricyclics, they are not sufficient for an accurate interpretation. It is necessary to test the reproducibility of data from tianeptine studies with other antidepressant drugs. In addition, it is necessary to support the experimental animal data with clinical trials. Neuroplasticity studies in humans were unable to go beyond morphological studies examining hippocampal formation and other important brain structures using magnetic resonance imaging techniques. It is certain that the development of non-invasive techniques that permit efficient assessment of central elements related to neuroplasticity in humans and comparison of these studies with clinical ones will herald a new era in the diagnosis and treatment of brain diseases.

References

Abraham, W.C., Dragunow, M., Tate W.P. (1991). The role of immediate early genes in the stabilization of long-term potentiation. *Mol. Neurobiol.* 5: 297-314.

Abumaria, N., Rygula, R., Hiemke, C., Fuchs, E., Havemann-Reinecke, U., Ruther, E., Flugge, G. (2007). Effect of chronic citalopram on serotonin-related and stress-regulated genes in the dorsal raphe nucleus of the rat. *Eur. Neuropsychopharmacol.* 17: 417-429.

Alboni S, Benatti C, Capone G, Corsini D, Caggia F, Tascedda F, Mendelewicz J, Brunello N. (2010). Time-dependent effects of escitalopram on brain derived neurotrophic factor (BDNF) and neuroplasticity related targets in the central nervous system of rats. *Eur. J. Pharmacol.* 643: 180-187.

Alfonso, J., Pollevick, G.D., Van Der Hart, M.G., Flugge, G., Fuchs, E., Frasch, A.C. (2004). Identification of genes regulated by chronic psychosocial stress and antidepressant treatment in the hippocampus. *Eur. J. Neurosci.* 19: 659-666.

Alfonso, J., Frick, L.R., Silberman, D.M., Palumbo, M.L., Genaro, A.M., Frasch, A.C. (2006). Regulation of hippocampal gene expression is conserved in two species subjected to different stressors and antidepressant treatments. *Biol. Psychiatry* 59: 244-251.

Alici, T., Kayir, H., Aygoren, M.O., Saglam, E., Uzbay, IT. (2006). Discriminative stimulus properties of tianeptine: partial substitution by fluoxetine and 8-OH-DPAT. *Psychopharmacology* 183: 446-451.

Allen, S.J., MacGowan, S.H., Treanor, J.J., Feeney, R., Wicock, G.K., Dawbarn, D. (1991). Normal beta-NGF content in Alzheimer's disease cerebral cortex and hippocampus. *Neurosci. Lett.* 131: 135-139.

Allgulander, C., Hackett, D., Salinas, E. (2001). Venlafaxine extended release (ER) in the treatment of generalised anxiety disorder. Twenty-four-week placebo-controlled dose-ranging study. *Br. J. Psychiatry* 179:15-22.

Angelucci, F., Mathe, A.A., Aloe, L. (2004). Neurotrophic factors and CNS disorders: finding in rodent models of depression and schizophrenia. Prog. Brain Res 46: 151-165.

Ansseau, M. (1988). *Les antidépresseurs. Méd. et Hyg.* 46: 2314-2321.

Ansseau, M. (1993). The paradox of tianeptine. *Eur. Psychiat.* 8 (Suppl. 2): 89S-93S.

Aprison, M.H., Hintgen, J.N., Nagayama, H. (1982). Testing a new theory of depression with an animal model; neurochemical-behavioral evidence for postsynaptic serotonergic receptor involvement. In: Langer, S.Z., Takahashi, R., Segawa, T., Briley, M. (Eds.), *New Vistas in Depression*, New york, Pergamon Press, pp.171-178.

Armstrong, R.C., Montminy, M.R. (1993). Transsynaptic control of gene expression. *Annu. Rev. Neurosci.* 16: 17-29.

Aydemir, C., Yalcin, E.S., Aksaray, S., Kisa, C., Yildirim, S.G., Uzbay, T., Goka, E. (2006). Brain-derived neurotrophic factor (BDNF) changes in the serum of depressed women. *Prog. Neuropsychopharmacol Biol. Psychiatry*, 30: 1256-1260.

Backman, C., Rose, G.M., Bartus, R.T., Hoffer, B.J., Mufson, E.J., Granholm, A.C. (1997). Carrier mediated delivery of NGF: Alterations in basal forebrain neurons in aged rats revealed using antibodies against low and high affinity NGF receptors. *J. Comp. Neurol.* 387: 1-11.

Ballarin, M., Emfors, P., Lindefors, N., Persson, H. (1991). Hippocampal damage and kainic acid injection induce a rapid increase in mRNA in the rat brain. *Exp. Neurol.* 114: 35-43.

Barbaccia, M.L., Gandolfi, O., Chuang, D.M., Costa, E. (1983). Modulation of neuronal serotonin uptake by a putative endogenous ligand of imipramine recognition sites. *Proc. Natl. Acad. Sci. USA* 80:5134-5138.

Biebl, M., Cooper, C.M., Winkler, J., Kuhn, H.G. (2000). Analysis of neurogenesis and programmed cell death reveals a self-renewing capacity in the adult rat brain. *Neurosci. Lett.* 291: 17-20.

Bird, E.D., Spokes, E.G., Iversen, L.L. (1979). Brain norepinephrine and dopamine in schizophrenia. *Science* 204: 93-94.

Birken, D.L., Oldendorf, W.H. (1989). N-acetyl-L-aspartic acid: a literature review of a compound prominent in 1H-NMR spectroscopy studies of the brain. *Neurosci. Biobehav. Rev.* 13: 23-31.

Blair, H.T., Schafe, G.E., Bauer, E.P., Rodrigues, S.M., LeDoux, J.E. (2001). Synaptic plasticity in the lateral amygdala: a cllular hypothesis of fear conditioning. *Learn Mem* 8: 229-242.

Bondy, B. (2002). Pathophysiology of depression and mechanisms of treatment. Dialogues in *Clinical Neuroscience*. 4: 7-20.

Boyer, P. (2000). Do anxiety and depression have a common pathophysiological mechanism? *Acta Psychiatr Scand* (Suppl. 406): 24-29.

Brand, A., Richter-Landsberg, C., Leibfritz, D. (1993). Multinuclear NMR studies on the energy metabolism of glial and neuronal cells. *Dev. Neurosci.* 15: 289-298.

Brewin, C.R. (2001). A cognitive neuroscience account of posttraumatic stress disorder and its treatment. *Behav. Res. Ther* 39: 373-393.

Brown, E.S., Rush, A.J., McEwen, B.S. (1999). Hippocampal remodelling and damage by corticosteroids: implications for mood disorders. *Neuropharmacology* 21: 474-484.

Brown, R.A.M., McKim, W.A. (2000). Neurophysiology, neurotransmitters, and the nervous system. In: McKim WA (Ed.), *Drugs and Behavior, An Introduction to Behavioral Pharmacology*. Printice Hall, New Jersey, pp. 56-81.

Brunello, N., Riva, M., Volterra, A., Racagni, G. (1987) Effect of some tricyclic and non tricyclic antidepressants on [3H] imipramine binding and serotonin uptake in rat cerebral cortex after prolonged treatment. *Fundam Clin. Pharmacol.* 1: 327-333.

Bunney, W.E., Davis, J.M. (1965). Norepinephrine in depressive reactions. *Arch. Gen. Psychiatry* 13: 483-494.

Burghardt, N.S., Sullivan, G.M., McEwen, B.S., Gorman, J.M., LeDoux, J.E. (2004). The selective serotonin reuptake inhibitor citalopram increases fear after acute treatment but reduces fear with chronic treatment: a comparison with tinaeptine. *Biol. Psychiatry* 55: 1171-1178.

Cahill, L. (2000). Neurobiological mechanisms of emotionally influenced long-term memory. *Prog. Brain Res.* 126: 29-37.

Cameron, H.A., McEwen, B.S., Gould, E. (1995). Regulation of adult neurogenesis by excitatory input and NMDA receptor activation in the dentate gyrus. *J. Neurosci.* 15: 4687-4692.

Carvey, P.M. (1998). *Drug Action in the Central Nervous System*. Oxford University Press, New York.

Castrén, E. (2005). Is mood chemistry? *Nature Rev.* 6: 241-246.

Ceyhan, M., Kayir, M., Uzbay, I.T. (2005). Investigation of the effects of tianeptine and fluoxetine on pentylenetetrazole-induced seizures in rats. *J. Psychiatric Res.* 39: 191-196.

Chang YC, Tzeng SF, Yu L, Huang AM, Lee HT, Huang CC, Ho CJ. (2006). Early-life fluoxetine exposure reduced functional deicits after hypoxic-ischemia brain injury in rat pups. *Neurobiol. Dis.* 24: 101-113.

Chao, M., Casaccia-Bonnefil, P., Carter, B., Chittka, A., Kong, H., Yoon, S.O. (1998). Neurotrophin receptors: mediators of life and death Brain res. *Brain res. Rev.* 26: 295-301.

Chao, M.V., Hempstead, B.L. (1995). P75 and Trk: a two-receptor system. *Trends Neurosci.* 18: 321-326.

Chaouloff, F. (1993). Psychopharmacological interactions between stress hormones and central serotonergic systems. *Brain Res. Rev.* 18: 1-32.

Chapman, P.F., Ramsay, M.F., Krezel, W., Knevett, S.G. (2003). Synaptic plasticity in the amygdala: comparisons with hippocampus. *Ann. NY Acad. Sci.* 985: 114-124.

Chen, G., Rajkowska, G., Du, F., Seraji-Bozorgzad, N., Manji, H.K. (2000). Enhancement of hippocampal neurogenezis by lithium. *J. Neurochem.* 75: 1729-1734.

Cotman,. CW., Nieto-Sampedro, M. (1984). Cell biology of synaptic plasticity. *Science* 225: 1287-1294.

Cowen, P.J. (1998). Pharmacological challenge tests and brain serotonergic function in depression during SSRI treatment. In: Briley, M., Montgomery, S. (Eds.), *Antidepressant Therapy,* Martin Dunitz Ltd, London, pp. 175-189.

Cutler, M.G., Rodgers, R.J., Jackson, J.E. (1997). Behavioural effects in mice of subchronic buspirone, ondansetron and tianeptine. I. Social interactions. *Pharmacol. Biochem. Behav.* 56: 287-293.

Czéh, B., Michaelis, T., Watanabe, T., Frahm, J., de Biurrun, G., van Kampen, M., Bartolomucci, A., Fuchs, E. (2001) Stress-induced changes in cerebral metabolites, hippocampal volume, and cell proliferation are prevented by antidepressant treatment with tianeptine. *Proc. Natl. Acad. Sci. USA* 98: 12796-12801.

Czéh, B., Welt, T., Fischer A.K., Erhardt, A., Schmitt W., Muller, M. (2002). Chronic psychosocial stress and concomitant repetitive transcranial magnetic stimulation: effects on stress hormone levels and adult hippocampal neurogenesis. *Biol. Psychiatry* 52: 1057-1065.

Defrance, R., Marey, C., Kamoun, A. (1988). Antidepressant and anxiolytic activities of tianeptine: an overview of clinical trials. *Clin. Neuropharmacol.* 11 (Suppl. 2): 74-82.

Delgado, P.L., Moreno, F.A., Potter, R., Gelenberg, A.J. (1998). Norepinephrine and serotonin in antidepressant action: evidence from neurotransmitter depletion studies. In: Briley, M., Montgomery, S. (Eds.), *Antidepressant Therapy*, Martin Dunitz Ltd, London, pp. 141-161.

Den Boer, J.A., Westenberg, H.G.M. (1988). Effect of a serotonin and noradrenaline uptake inhibitor in panic disorder; a double-blind comparative study with fluvoxamine and maprotiline. *Int. Clin. Psychopharmacol.* 3: 59-74.

Diamond, D.M., Rose, G.M. (1994). Stress impairs. LTP and hippocampal-dependent memory. *Ann. NY Acad Sci.* 746: 411-414.

Diamond, D.M., Campbell, A., Park, C.R., Vouimba, R-M. (2004). Preclinical research on stress, memory, and the brain in the development of pharmacotherapy for depression. *Eur. Neuropsychopharmacol.* 14 (Suppl. 5) : S491-S495.

Dowlatshahi, D., MacQuenn, G.M., Wang, J.F., Young, LT. (1998). Increased temporal cortex CREB concentrations and antidepressant treatment in major depression. *Lancet* 352: 1754-1755.

Dragunow, M., Robertson, G.S., Faull, R.L.M., Robertson, H.A., Jansen, K. (1990). D2 dopamine receptor antagonists induce Fos and related proteins in rat striatal neurons. *Neuroscience* 37: 287-294.

Dubovsky, S.L., Thomas, M. (1995). Beyond specifity: effects of serotonin and serotonergic treatments on psychobiological dysfunction. *J. Psychosom. Res.* 39: 429-444.

Duman, R.S. (1998). Novel therapeutic approaches beyond the 5-HT receptor. *Biol. Psychiatry* 44: 324-335.

Duman, R.S., Nakagawa, S., Malberg, J. (2001). Regulation of adult neurogenezis by antidepressant treatment. *Neuropsychopharmacology* 25: 836-844.

Duman, R.S. (2002). Pathophysiology of depression: the concept of synaptic plasticity. *Eur. Psychiatry* 17 (Suppl. 3): 306-310.

Duman, R.S. (2004). Neural plasticity: consequences of stress and actions of antidepressant treatment. *Dialogues in Clinical Neuroscienve – Neuroplasticity.* 6: 157-169.

Eisch, A.J. (2002). Adult neurogenesis: implications for psychiatry. *Prog. Brain Res.* 138: 315-342.

Ericksson, P.S., Perfilieva, E., Björk-Eriksson, T., Alborn, A., Nordberg, C., Peterson, D.A., Gage, F.H. (1998). Neurogenezis in the adult human hippocampus. *Nature Medicine* 4: 1313-1317.

Fattaccini, C.M., Bolanos-Jimenez, F., Gozlan, H., Hamon, M. (1990). Tianeptine stimulates uptake of 5-hydroxytryptamine in vivo in the rat brain. *Neuropharmacology* 29: 1-8.

Feldman, R.S., Meyer, J.S., Qenzer, L.F. (1997). Principles of Neuropsychopharmacology. Sinauer Associates Inc., Sunderland, Massachusetts, pp. 58-491.

Fichter, M.M., Narrow, W.E., Roper, M.T., Rehm, J., Elton, M., Rae, D.S., Locke, B.Z., Regier, D.A. (1996). Prevalance of mental illness in Germany and the United States: comparison of the Upper Bavarian Study and the Epidemiologic Catchment Area Program. *J. Nerv. Ment Dis*, 184: 598-606.

Forstermann, U., Gorsky, L.D., Pollock, J.S., Schmidt, H.H., Heler, M., Murad, F. (1990). Regional distribution of EDRF/NO-synthesizing enzyme(s) in rat brain. *Biochem. Biophys. Res. Commun* 168: 727-732.

Fossati, P., Harvey, P.O., Le Bastard, G., Ergis, A.M., Jouvent, R., Allilaire, J.F. (2004). Verbal memory performance of patients with a first depressive episode and patients with unipolar and bipolar recurrent depression. *J. Psychiatr. Res.* 38: 137-144.

Foy, M.R., Stanton, M.E., Levine, S., Thompson, R.F. (1987). Behavioral stress impairs long-term potentiation in rodent hippocampus. *Behav. Neural. Biol.* 48: 138-149.

Frechila D, Otano A, Del Rio J. (1998). Effect of chronic antidepressant treatment on transcription factor binding activity in rat hippocampus and frontal cortex. *Prog. Neuropsychopharmacol. Biol. Psychiatry* 22: 787-802.

Chang, Y.C., Tzeng, S.F., Yu, L., Huang, A.M., Lee, H.T., Huang, C.C., Ho, C.J. (1998). Effects of chronic antidepressant treatment on transcription factor binding activity in rat hippocampus and frontal cortex. *Prog. Neuropsychopharmacol. Biol. Psychiatry* 22: 787-802.

Fuchs, E., Gould, E. (2000). Mini-review: in vivo neurogenesis in the adult brain: regulation and functional implications. *Eur. J. Neurosci* 12: 2211-2214.

Fuchs, E., Czéh, B., Michaelis, T., de Biurrun, G., Watanabe, T., Frahm, J. (2002). Synaptic plasticity and tianeptine: structural regulation. *Eur. Psychiatry* 17 (Suppl. 3): 311-317.

Fuchs, E., Czéh, B., Kole, M.H.P., Michaelis, T., Lucassen, P.L. (2004). Alterations of neuroplasticity in depression: the hippocampus and beyond. *Eur. Neuropsychopharmacol.* 14: S481-S490.

Fuchs, E. (2009). Neuroplasticity – A new approach to the pathophysiology of depression. In: Costa e Silva JA, Macher JP, Olié JP (Eds.), *Neuroplasticity. New Biochemicakl Mechanism.* Current Medicine Group, London, pp. 1-12.

Gall, C.M., Gold, S.J., Isackson, P.J., Seroogy, K.B. (1992). Brain derived neurotrophic factor and neurotrophin -3 mRNAs are expressed in ventral midbrain regions containing dopaminergic neurons. *Mol. Cell Neurosci.* 3: 56-63.

Garattini, S., Giacolone, E., Valzelli, L. (1967). Isolation, agressiveness and brain 5-hydroxytriptamine turnover. *J. Pharm. Pharmacol.* 19: 338-339.

Garthwaite, J., Garthwaite, G., Palmer, R.M., Moncada, S. (1989). NMDA receptor activation induces nitric oxide synthesis from arginine in rat brain slices. *Eur. J. Pharmacol.* 172: 413-416.

Garthwaite, J. (1991). Glutamate, nitric oxide and cell-cell signalling in the nervous system. *Trends Neurosci.* 14: 60-67.

Garzon, J., del Rio, J. (1981). Hypersensitivity induced in rats by long tern isolation: Further studies on a new animal model for the detection of antidepressants. *Eur. J. Pharmacol.* 74: 287-294.

Goggi, J., Pullar, I.A., Carney, S.L., Bradford, H.F. (2002). Modulation of neurotransmitter release induced by brain-derived neurotrophic factor in rat brain striatal slices in vitro. *Brain Res.* 941: 34-42.

Goldberg, H.L., Finnerty, R.J. (1979). The comparative efficacy of buspirone and diazepam in the treatment of anxiety. *Am. J. Psychiatry* 136: 1184-1187.

Gould, E., McEwen, B.S., Tanapat, P., Galea, L.A., Fuchs, E. (1997). Neurogenezis in the dentate gyrus of the adult tree shrew is regulated by psychosocial stress and NMDA receptor activation. *J. Neurosci.* 17: 2492-2498.

Gould, E., Tanapat, P., McEwen, B.S., Flugge, G., Fuchs, E. (1998). Proliferation of granule cell precursors in the dentate gyrus of adult monkeys is diminished by stress. *Proc. Natl. Acad. Sci. USA* 95: 3168-3171.

Gould, E. (1999). Serotonin and hippocampal neurogenesis. *Neuropsychopharmacology* 21: 46S-51S.

Gross, C.G. (2000). Neurogenesis in the adult brain: death of a dogma. *Nat. Rev. Neurosci.* 1: 67-73.

Gören, M.Z., Arıcıoğlu-Kartal, F., Yurdun, T., Uzbay, I.T. (2001). Investigation of extracellular L-citrulline concentration in the striatum during alcohol withdrawal in rats. *Neurochem. Res.*, 26: 1327-1333.

Graybiel, A.M., Moratalla, R., Robertson, H.A. (1990). Amphetamine and cocaine induce drug-specific activation of the c-fos gene in striosome-matrix compartments and limbic subdivisions of the striatum. *Proc. Natl. Acad. Sci. USA* 87: 6912-6916.

Guelfi, J.D., Pichot, P., Dreyfus, J.F. (1989). Efficacy of tianeptine in anxious-depressed patients. Results of a controlled multicentre trial versus amitriptyline, *Neuropsychobiology* 1: 41-48.

Heasley, L.E., Storey, B., Fanger, G.R., Butterfield, L., Zamarripa, J., Blumberg, D., Maue, R.A. (1996). GTPase-deficient G alpha 16 and G alpha q induce PC12 cell differentiation and persistent activation of cJun NH2-terminal kinases. *Mol. Cell Biol.* 16: 648-656.

Heine, V.M., Malsam, S., Zareno, J., Joëls, M., Lucassen, P.J. (2004). Supressed proliferation and apoptotic changes in the rat dentate gyrus after acute and chronic stress are reversible. *Eur. J. Neurosci.* 19: 131-144.

Hindmarch, I. (2002). Beyond the monoamine hypothesis: mechanisms, molecules and methods. *Eur. Psychiatry* 17 (Suppl. 3): 294-299.

Hoehn-Saric, R. (1982). Neurotransmitters in anxiety. *Arch. Gen. Psychiatry* 39:735-742.

Hyman, S.E., Nestler, E.J. (1996). Initiation and adaptation: A paradigm for understanding psychotrophic drug action. *Am. J. Psychiatry* 153: 151-162.

Ip, N.Y., Ibanez, C.F., Nye, S.H., McClain, J., Jones, P.F., Gies, D.R., Belluscio, L., Le Beau, M.M., Espinoza III, R., Squinto, S.P. (1992). Mammalian neurotrophin-4: structure, chromosomal localization, tissue distribution, and receptor specificity. *Proc. Natl. Acad. Sci. USA* 89: 3060-3064.

Jacobs, B.L., Praag, H., Gage, F.H. (2000). Adult brain neurogenesis and psychiatry: a novel theory of depression. *Mol. Psychiatry* 5: 262-269.

Kaplan, D.R., Miller, F.D. (2000). Neurotrophin signal transduction in the nervous system. *Curr. Opin. Neurobiol.* 10: 381-391.

Kato, G., Weitsch, A.F. (1988). Neurochemical profile of tianeptine, a new antidepressant drug. *Clin. Neuropharmacol.* 11 (Suppl. 2): S43-S50.

Kato, T., Inubushi, T., Kato, N. (1998). Magnetic resonance spectroscopy in affective disorders. *J. Neuropsychiatry Clin. Neurosci.* 10: 133-147.

Katoh-Semba, R., Asano, T., Ueda, H., Morishita, R., Takeuchi, I.K., Inaguma, Y, Kato, K. (2002). *Faseb. J.* 16: 1328-1330.

Kempermann, G., Kronenberg, G. (2003). Depressed new neurons?- Adult hippocampal neurogenezis and a cellular plasticity hypothesis of major depression. *Biol. Psychiat.* 54: 499-503.

Kennedy, S.H., Lam, R.W., Nutt, D.J., Thase, M.E. (2004). Treating Depression Effectively. *Applying Clinical Guidelines.* Martin Dunitz Ltd, London, pp. 47-55.

Kiba, H., Jayaraman, A. (1994). Nicotine-induced c-fos expression in the striatum is mediated mostly by dopamine D1 receptor and is dependent on NMDA stimulation. *Mol. Brain Res.* 23: 1-13.

Kim, J.J., Diamond, D.M. (2002). The stressed hippocampus, synaptic plasticity and lost memories. *Nat. Rev. Neurosci.* 3: 453-462.

Kim, Y.K., Lee, H.P., Won, S.D., Park, E.Y., Lee, H.Y., Lee, B.H., Lee, S.W., Yoon, D., Han, C., Kim, D.J., Choi, S.H. (2007). Low plasma BDNF is associated with suicidal behavior in major depression. *Prog. Neuropsychopharmacol. Biol. Psychiatry* 31: 78-85.

Kole, M.H.P., Swan, L., Fuchs, E. (2002). The antidepressant tianeptine persistently modulates glutamate receptor currents of the hippocampal CA3 commissural associational synapse in chronically stressed rats. *Eur. J. Neurosci.* 16: 807-816.

Konradi, C., Cole, R.L., Heckers, S., Hyman, S.E. (1994). Amphetamine regulates gene expression in rat striatum via transcription factor CREB. *J. Neurosci.* 14: 5623-5634.

Kuhn, H.G., Palmer, T.D., Fuchs, E. (2001). Adult neurogenesis: a compensatory mechanism for neuronal damage. *Eur. Arch. Psychiatry Clin. Neurosci.* 251: 152-158.

Kuipers, S.D., Trentani, A., ter Horst, G.J., den Boer, JA. (2005). Looking beyond the receptor: Molecular biological approaches to antidepressant therapy. In: Den Boer, J.A., George, M.S., ter Horst, G.J. (Eds.), *Current and Future Developments in Psychopharmacology.* Benecke NI, Amsterdam, pp. 83-102.

Landfield, P.W. (1994). Increased hippocampal Ca2+ channel activity in brain aging and dementia. Hormonal and pharmacological modulation. *Ann. NY Acad. Sci.* 747: 351-364.

Leonard, B.E. (1998). Animal models of depression. In: Briley, M., Montgomery, S. (Eds.), *Antidepressant Therapy*, Martin Dunitz Ltd, London, pp. 87-109.

Lepine, J.P., Gastpar, M., Mendelwicz, J., Tylee, A. (1997). The prevalence of depression in the community; the first pan-European study DEPRES

(Depression Research in European Society). *Int. Clin. Psychopharmacol.*, 12: 19-29.

Leverenz, J.B., Wilkinson, C.W., Wamble, M., Corbin, S., Grabber, J.E., Raskind, M.A. (1999). Effect of chronic high-dose exogenous cortisol on hippocampal neuronal number in aged nonhuman primates. *J. Neurosci.* 19: 2356-2361.

Levin, G.R., Barde, Y.A. (1996). Physiology of the neurotrophins. *Annu. Rev. Neurosci.* 19: 289-317.

Liu, J., Nickolenko, J., Sharp, F.R. (1994). Morphine induces c-fos and junB in striatum and nucleus accumbens via D1 and N-methyl-D-aspartate receptors. *Proc. Natl. Acad. Sci. USA* 91: 8537-8541.

Lõo, H., Saiz-Ruiz, J., Costa e Silva, J.A., Ansseau, M., Herrington, R., Vaz-Serra, A., Dilling, H., De Risio, S. (2001). Efficacy and safety of tianeptine in the treatment of depressive disorders in comparison with fluoxetine. *Hum. Psychopharmacol.* 16 (Suppl. 1): S31-S38.

Lowy, M.T., Gault, L., Yamamato, B.K. (1993). Adrenalectomy attenuates stress-induced elevations in extracellular glutamate concentrations in the hippocampus. *J. Neurochem.* 61: 1957-1960.

Lowy, M.T., Wittenberg, L., Yamamto, B.K. (1995). Effects of acute stress in hippocampal glutamate levels and spectrin preteolysis in young and aged rats. *J. Neurochem.* 65: 268-274.

Lucassen, P.J., Muller, M.B., Holsboer, F., Bauer, J., Holtrop, A., Wouda, J., Hoogendijk, W.J., De Kloet, E.R., Swaab, D.F. (2001). Hippocampal apoptosis in major depression is a minor event and absent from subareas at risk for glucocorticoid overexposure. *Am. J. Pathol.* 158: 453-68.

Lucassen, P.J., Fuchs, E., Czéh, B. (2004). Antidepressant treatment with tianeptine reduces apopitosis in hippocampal dentate gyrus and temporal cortex. *Biol. Psychiatry* 55: 789-796.

Lupien, S.J., McEwen, B.S. (1997). The acute effects of corticosteroids on cognition: integration of animal and human model studies. *Brain Res. Rev.* 24: 1-27.

Maas, J.W., Fawcett, J., Dekimejian, H. (1968). 3-methoxy-4-hydoxy-phenylglycol (MHPG) excretion in depressive patients. *Arch. Gen. Psychiatry* 19: 129-134.

Madsen, T.M., Trechow, A., Bengzon, J., Bolwig, T.G., Lindvall, O., Tingstrom, A. (2000). Increased neurogenezis in a model of electroconvulsive therapy. *Biol. Psychiatry* 47: 1043-1049.

Magarinos, A.M., McEwen, B.C. (1995a). Stress-induced athrophy of apical dendrites of hippocampal CA3c neurons: comparison of stressors. *Neuroscience* 69: 83-88.

Magarinos, A.M., McEwen, B.C. (1995b). Stress-induced athrophy of apical dendrites of hippocampal CA3c neurons: involvement of glucocorticoid secretion and excitatory amino acid receptors. *Neuroscience* 69: 89-98.

Magarinos, A.M., McEwen, B.S., Flugge, G., Fuchs, E. (1996). Chronic psychosocial stress causes apical dentritic athrophy of hippocampal CA3 pyramidal neurons in subordinate tree shrews. *J Neurosci* 16: 3534-3540.

Magarinos, A.M., Verdugo, J.M., McEwen, B.S. (1997). Chronic stress alters synaptic terminal structure in hippocampus. *Proc. Natl. Acad. Sci. USA* 94: 14002-14008.

Magarinos, A.M., Deslandes, A., McEwen, B.S. (1999). Effects of antidepressants and benzodiazepine treatments on the dendritic structure of CA3 pyramidal neurons after chronic stress. *Eur. J. Pharmacol.* 371: 113-122.

Maghaddam, B., Boliano, M.L., Stein-Behrens, B., Sapolsky, R. (1994). Glucocorticoids mediate the stress-induced extracellular accumulation of glutamate. *Brain Res.* 655: 251-254.

Maisonpierre, P.C., Le Beau, M.M., Espinosa III, R., Ip, N.Y., Belluscio, L., de la Monte, S.M., Squinto, S., Furth, M.E., Yancopoulos, G.D. (1991). Human and rat brain-derived neurotrophic factor and neurotrophin-3 : gene structures, distributions, and chromosomal localizations. *Genomics* 10: 558-568.

Malberg, J.E., Eisch, A.J., Nestler, E.J., Duman, R.S. (2000). Chronic antidepressant treatment increases neurogenezis in adult rat hippocampus. *J. Neurosci.* 20: 9104-9110.

Mailleux, P., Verslype, M., Preud'homme, X., Vanderhaeghen, J-J. (1994). Activation of multiple transcription factor genes by tetrahidrocannabinol in rat forebrain. *Neuroreport* 5: 1265-1268.

Manji, H.K., Duöam, R.S. (2001). Impairments of neuroplasticity and cellular resilience in severe modd disorders: implications for the development of novel therapeutics. *Psychopharmacol. Bull.* 35: 5-49.

Manji, H.K., Quiroz, J.A., Sporn, J., Payne, J.L., Denicoff, K.A., Gray, N., Zarate, Jr., C.A, Charney, D.S. (2003). Enhancing neuronal plasticity and cellular resilience to develop novel improved therapeutics for difficult-to-treat depression. *Biol. Psychiatry* 53: 707-742.

Mann, J.J., Brown, R.P. (1985). A clinical perspective on the role of neurotransmitters in mental disorders. *Hospital and Community Psychiatry* 36: 141-150.

Maren, S., Fanselow, M.S. (1995). Synaptic plasticity in the basolateral amygdala induced by hippocampal formation stimulation in vivo. *J. Neurosci.* 15: 7548-7564.

Marsden, C.D. (1982). Neurotransmitters and CNS disease-Basal ganglia disease. *Lancet ii:* 1141-1146.

Marvanová, M., Lakso, M., Pirhonen, J., Nawa, H., Wong, G., Castrén, E. (2001). The neuroprotective agent memantine induces brain-derived neurotrophic factor and trkB receptor expression in rat brain. *Mol. Cell Neurosci.* 18: 247-258.

Mason, S.T., Fibiger, H.C. (1979). Anxiety: The locus coeruleus disconnection. *Life Sci* 25: 2141-2147.

McAllister, A.K., Katz, L.C., Lo, D.C. (1999). Neurotrophins and synaptic plasticity. *Annu. Rev. Neurosci.* 22: 295-318.

McEwen, B.S., Weiss, J.M., Schwartz, L.S. (1968). Selective retention of corticosterone by limbic structures in rat brain. *Nature* 220: 911-912.

McEwen, B.S., Weiss, J.M. (1970). The uptake and action of corticosterone: regional and subcellular studies on rat brain. *Prog. Brain Res.* 32: 200-212.

McEwen, B.S., Sapolsky, R.M. (1995). Stress and cognitive function. *Curr. Opin. Neurobiol.* 5: 205-216.

McEwen, B.S., Conrad, C.D., Kuroda, Y., Frankfurt, M., Magarinos, A.M., McKittrick, C. (1997). Prevention of stress-induced morphological and cognitive consequences. *Eur. Neuropsychopharmacol.* 7 (Suppl. 3) : S323-S328.

McEwen, B.S. (1999a). Stress and the aging hippocampus. *Front Endocrinol.* 20: 49-70.

McEwen, B.S. (1999b). Stress and hippocampal plasticity. *Annu. Rev. Neurosci.* 22: 105-122.

McEwen, B.S., Magarinos, A.M., Reagan, L.P. (2002). Structural plasticity and tianeptine: cellular and molecular targets. *Eur. Psychiatry* 17 (Suppl. 3): 318-330.

McEwen, B.S. (2004). Structural plasticity of the adult brain: how animal models help us understand brain changes in depression and systemic disorders related to depression. *Dialogues in Clinical Science – Neuroplasticity* 6: 119-133.

McKim, W.A. (2000). *Drugs and Behavior: An Introduction to Behavioral Pharmacology*, Fourth Edition, Prentice-Hall Inc., New Jersey, pp. 26-347.

Menini, T., Mocaer, E., Garattini, S. (1987). Tianeptine, a selective enhancer of serotonin uptake in rat brain. *Naunyn-Schmiedeberg's Arch. Pharmacol.* 336: 478-482.

Minneman, K.P. (1991). Pharmacological organization of the CNS. In: Wingard LB, Brody TM, Larner J, Schwartz A (Eds.), *Human Pharmacology, Molecular to Clinical.* Wolfe Publishing Limited, London, pp. 299-341.

Mizoguchi, K., Kunishita, T., Chui, D.H., Tabira, T. (1992). Stress induces neuronal death in the hippocampus of castrated rats. *Neurosci. Lett.* 138: 157-160.

Moghaddam, B., Bolinao, M.L., Stein-Behrens, B., Sapolsky, R. (1994). Glucocorticoids mediate the stress-induced extracellular accumulation of glutamate. *Brain Res.* 655: 251-254.

Moghaddam, B. (2002). Stress activation of glutamate neurotransmission in the prefrontal cortex: implications for dopamine-associated psychiatric disorders. *Biol. Psychiatry* 51: 775-787.

Moncada, S., Higgs, A. (1993). The L-arginine-nitric oxide pathway. *N. Engl. J. Med.* 329: 2002-2012.

Moncada, S., Higgs, A., Furchgott, R. (1997). XIV. International union of pharmacology nomenclature in nitric oxide research. *Pharmacol. Rev.* 49: 137-142.

Morgan, J.I., Curran, T. (1989). Stimulus-transcription coupling in neurons: Role of cellular immediate-early genes. *Trends Neurosci.* 12: 459-462.

Morinobu S, Russel DS, Sugawara S, Takahashi M, Fujimaki K. (2000). Regulation of phosphorylation of cyclic AMP response element-binding protein by paroxetine treatments. *Clin. Neuropharmacol.* 23: 106-109.

Mostany R, Valdizan EM, Pazos A. (2008). A role for nuclear beta-catenin in SNRI antidepressant-induced hippocampal cell proliferation. *Neuropharmacology* 55: 18-26.

Mukobata, S., Hibino, T., Sugiyama, A., Urano, Y., Inatomi, A., Kanai, Y., Endo, H., Tashiro, F. (2002). M6a acts as a nerve growth factor-gated Ca(2+) channel in neuronal differentiation. *Biochem. Biophys. Res. Commun.* 297: 722-728.

Myers, M.P., Murphy, M.B., Landreth, G. (1994). The dual-specificity CLK kinase induces neuronal differentiation of PC12 cells. *Mol. Cell Biol.* 14: 6954-6961.

Nagayama, H., Hinntgen, J.N., Aprison, M.H. (1980). Pre- and post-synaptic serotonergic manipulations in an animal model of depression. *Pharmacol. Biochem. Behav.* 13: 575-579.

Nakajima, S., Daval, J-C., Morgan, P.F., Post, R.M., Marangos, P.J. (1989). Adenosinergic modulation of caffeine-induced c-fos mRNA expression in mouse brain. *Brain Res.* 501: 307-314.

Natthanson, J.A. (1977). Cyclic nucleotides and nervous system function. *Physiol. Rev.* 57: 157-256.

Nibuya, M., Morinobu, S., Duman, R.S. (1995). Regulation of BDNF and trkB mRNA in rat brain by chronic electroconvulsive seizure and antidepressant drug treatments. *J. Neurosci.* 15: 7539-7547.

Nibuya, M., Nestler, E.J., Duman, R.S. (1996). Chronic antidepressant administration increases the expression of cAMP response element binding protein (CREB) in rat hippocampus. *J. Neurosci.* 16: 2365-2372.

Ninan, P.T. (1999). The functional anatomy, neurochemistry, and pharmacology of anxiety. *J. Clin. Psychiatry* 60 (Suppl. 22): 12-17.

Ohl, F., Michaelis, T., Vollmann-Honsdorf, G.K., Kirschbaum, C., Fuchs, E. (2000). Effect of chronic psychosocial stress and long-term cortisol treatment on hippocampus-mediated memory and hippocampal volume: a plot study in tree shrews. *Psychoneuroendocrinology* 25: 357-363.

Olivier, B., van Wijngaarden, I., Soudijn, W. (2000). 5-HT3 receptor antagonists and anxiety; a preclinical and clinical review. *Eur. Neuropsychopharmacol.* 10: 77-95.

Ozawa, H., Saito, T., Takahata, N. (Eds.). (1998). *Signal Transduction in Affective Disorders*. Springer, Tokyo.

Pacher, P., Kohegyi, E., Kecskemeti, V., Furst, S. (2001). Current trends in the development of new antidepressants. *Curr. Med. Chem.* 8: 89-100.

Parker, K.J., Schatzberg, A.F., Lyons, D.M. (2003). Neuroendocrine aspects of hypercortisolism in major depression. *Horm. Behav.* 43: 60-66.

Pavlides, C., Watanabe, Y., Magarinos, A.M., McEwen, B.S. (1995). Opposing roles of type I and type II adrenal steroid receptors in hippocampal long-term potentiation. *Neuroscience* 68: 387-394.

Pham, K., Nacher, J., Hof, P.R., McEwen, B.S. (2003). Repeated restraintstress suppresses neurogenesis and induces biphasic PSA-NCAM expression in the adult rat dentate gyrus. *Eur. J. Neurosci.* 17: 879-886.

Pineyro, G., Blier, P.A. (1999). Autoregulation of serotonin neurons: role in antidepressant drug action. *Pharmacol. Rev.* 51: 533-591.

Plaisant, F., Dommergues, M.A., Spedding, M., Cecchelli, R., Brillaut, J., Kato, G., Munoz, C., Gressens, P. (2003). Neuroprotective properties of tianeptine : interactions with cytokines. *Neuropharmacology* 44: 801-809.

Poldrack, R.A., Gabrieli, J.D. (1997). Functional anatomy of long-term memory. *J. Clin. Neurophysiol.* 14: 294-310.

Popoli, M., Gennarelli, M., Racagni, G. (2002). Modulation of synaptic plasticity by stress and antidepressants. *Bipolar. Disord.* 4: 166-182.

Quitkin, F.M., Rabkin, J.G., Ross., D., McGrath, P.J. (1984). Duration of antidepressant drug treatment. What is an adequate trial? *Arch. Gen. Psychiatry* 41: 238-245.

Rang, H.P., Dale, M.M., Ritter, J.M. (1999). *Pharmacology,* 4th Edition, Churchill Livingstone, Edinburgh, pp. 483-538.

Reagan, L.P., Rosell, D.R., Wood, G.E., Spedding, M., Munoz, C., Rothstein, J., McEwen, B.S. (2004) Chronic restraint stress up-regulates GLT-1 mRNA and protein expression in the rat hippocampus: reversal by tianeptine. *Proc. Natl. Acad. Sci. USA* 101: 2197-2184.

Reagan LP, Hendry RM, Reznikov LR, Piroli GG, Wood GE, McEwen BS, Grillo CA. (2007). Tianeptine increases brain-derived neurotrophic factor expression in the rat amygdala. *Eur. J. Pharmacol.* 565: 68-75.

Reyntjens, A., Gelders, Y.G., Hoppenbrouwers, M.L. (1986). Thymosthenic effects of ritanserin (R55667), a centrally acting serotonin S2 receptor blocker. *Drug Dev. Res.* 8: 205-211.

Richelson, E. (2001). Pharmacology of antidepressants. *Mayo Clin. Proc.* 76: 511-527.

Rocher, C., Spedding, M., Munoz, C., Jay, T.M. (2004). Acute stress-induced changes in hippocampal/prefrontal circuits in rats: effects of antidepressants. *Cerabral. Cortex* 14: 224-229.

Rogan, M.T., Staubli, U.V., LeDoux, J.E. (1997). Fear conditioning induces associative long-term potentiation in the amygdala. *Nature* 390: 604-607.

Roseboom, P.H., Klein, D.C. (1995). Norepinephrine stimulation of pineal cyclic AMP response element-binding protein phosphorylation: primary role of a beta-adrenergic receptor/cyclic AMP mechanism. *Mol. Pharmacol.* 47: 439-449.

Rossor, M.N. (1982). Neurotransmitters and CNS disease – Demantia. *Lancet* *ii*: 1200-1204.

Saarelainen, T., Hendolin, P., Lucas, G., Koponen, E., Sairanen, M., MacDonald, E., Agerman, K., Haapasalo, A., Nawa, H., Aloyz, R., Ernfors, P., Castrén, E. (2003). Activation of the TrkB neurotrophin receptor is induced by antidepressant drugs and is required for antidepressant-induced behavioral effects. *J. Neurosci.*, 23: 349-357.

Sagar, S.M., Sharp, F.R. (1993). Early response genes as markers of neuronal activity and growth factor action. *Adv. Neurol.* 59: 273-284.

Sah, D.W.Y., Ossipov, M.H., Porreca, F. (2003). Neuropathic factors as novel therapeutics for neuropathic pain. *Nature Reviews* 2: 460-472.

Sala, M., Perez, J., Soloff, P., di Nemi, S.U., Caverzasi, E., Soares, J.C., Brambilla, P. (2004). Stress and hippocampus abnormalities in psychiatric disorders. *Eur. Neuropsychopharmacol.* 14: 393-405.

Sapolsky, R.M., Uno, H., Rebert, C.S., Finch, C.E. (1990). Hippocampal damage associated with prolonged glucocorticoid exposure in primates. *J. Neurosci.* 10: 2897-2902.

Sapolsky, R.M. (2000). Glucocorticoids and hippocampal atrophy in neuropsychiatric disorders. *Arch. Gen. Psychiatry* 57: 925-935.

Savas, H.A., Herken, H., Yurekli, M., Uz, E., Tutkun, H., Zoroglu, S.S., Ozen, M.E., Cengiz, B, Akyol, O. (2002). Possible role of nitric oxide and adrenomedullin in bipolar affective disorder. *Neuropsychobiology* 45: 57-61.

Scaccianoce, S., Del Bianco, P., Caricasole, A., Nicoletta, F., Catalini, A. (2003). Relationship between learning, stress and hippocampal brain-derived neurotrophic factor. *Neuroscience* 121: 825-828.

Schaaf, M.J., De Kloet, E.R., Vreugdenhil, E. (2000). Corticosterone effects on BDNF expression in the hippocampus. Implications for memory formation. *Stress* 3: 201-208.

Schildkraut, J.J. (1965). The catecholamine hypothesis of affective disorders: a review of supporting evidence. *Am. J. Psychiatry* 122: 509-522.

Schmidt, H.D., Duman, R.S. (2007). The role of neurotrophic factors in adult hippocampal neurogenezis, antidepressant treatments and animal models of depressive-like behavior. *Behav. Pharmacol.* 18: 391-418.

Scott, B.W., Wojtowicz, J.M., Burnham, W.M. (2000). Neurogenezis in the dentate gyrus of the rat following electroconvulsive shock seizures. *Exp. Neurol.* 165: 231-236.

Selye, H. (1976). Forty years of stress research: principal remaining problems and misconceptions. *Can. Med. Assoc. J.* 115: 53-56.

Sepinwall, J., Cook, L. (1980). Mechanisms of action of the benzodiazepines: Behavioral aspect. *Fed. Proc.* 39: 3024-3031.

Shamir, A., Agam, G., Belmaker, R.H. (2005). Neurogenesis and neuroprotection as new drug targets for bipolar disorder: a critical review. In: Den Boer, J,A,, George, M.S., ter Horst, G.J. (Eds.), *Current and*

Future Developments in Psychopharmacology. Benecke NI, Amsterdam, pp. 217-229.

Sheline, Y.I. (2000). 3D MRI studies of neuroanatomic changes in unipolar major depression: the role of stress and medical comorbidity. *Biol. Psychiatry* 48: 791-800.

Sheline, Y.I., Gado, M.H., Kraemer, H.C. (2003). Untreated depression and hippocampal volume loss. *Am. J. Psychiatry* 160: 1516-1518.

Shirayama, Y., Chen, A.C., Nakagawa, S., Russel, R.S., Duman, R.S. (2002). Brain derived neurotrophic factor produces antidepressant effects in behavioral models of depression. *J. Neurosci.* 22: 3251-3261.

Shoval, G., Weizman, A. (2005). The possible role of neurotrophins in the pathogenesis and therapy of schizophrenia. *Eur. Neuropsychopharmacol.* 15: 319-329.

Shu, S.Y., Wu, Y.M., Bao, X.M., Leonard, B. (2003). Interactions among memory-related centers in the brain. *J. Neurosci. Res.* 71: 609-616.

Snyder, S.H. (1982). Neurotransmitters and CNS disease – Schizophrenia. Lancet ii: 970-973.

Snyder, S.H., Bredt, D.S. (1992). Biological roles of nitric oxide. *Sci. Am.* May: 68-77.

Sousa, N., Lukoyanov, N.V., Madeira, M.D., Almeida, O.F., Paula-Barbosa, M.M. (2000). Reorganization of the morphology of hippocampal neuritis and synapses after stress-induced damage correlates with behavioral improvement. *Neuroscience* 97: 253-266.

Squire, L.R. (1992). Memory and hippocampus: a synthesis from findings with rats, monkeys, and humans. *Psychol. Rev.* 99: 195-231.

Stahl, S.M. (1996). *Essential Psychopharmacology.* Cambridge University Press, Cambridge, pp. 1-47.

Stahl, S.M. (2000). E*ssential Psychopharmacology. Neuroscientific Basis and Practical Applications.* Second Edition, Cambridge University Press, Cambridge.

Starkman, M.N., Giordani, B., Gebarski, S.S., Schteingart, D.E. (2003). Improvement in learning associated with increase in hippocampal formation volume. *Biol. Psychiat.* 53: 233-238.

Stein, L., Wise, D.C., Belluzi, J.D. (1975). Effects of benzodiazepines on central serotonergic mechanisms. *Adv. Biocehem. Psychopharmacol.* 10: 1-12.

Stein-Behrens, B.A., Lin, W.J., Sapolsky, R.M. (1994). Physiological elevations of glucocorticoids potentiate glutamate accumulation in the hippocampus. *J. Neurochem.* 63: 596-602.

Tardito D, Mesazzi L, Tiraboschi E, Mallei A, Racagni G, Popoli M. (2009). Early induction of CREB activation and CREB-regulating signalling by antidepressants. *Int. J. Neuropsychopharmacol.* 12: 1367-1381.

Thome, J., Sakai, N., Shin, K., Steffen, C., Zhang, Y.J., Impey, S., Storm, D., Duman, R.S. (2000). cAMP response element-mediated gene transcription is upregulated by chronic antidepressant treatment. *J. Neurosci.* 20: 4030-4036.

Uno, H., Tarara, R., Else, J.G., Suleman, M.A., Sapolsky, R.M. (1989). Hippocampal damage associated with prolonged and fatal stress in primates. *J. Neurosci.* 9: 1705-1711.

Urenjak, J., Willliams, S.R., Gadian, D.G., Noble, M. (1993). Proton nuclear magnetic resonance spectroscopy unambiguously idendifies different neural cell types. *J. Neurosci.* 13: 981-989.

Uzbay, I.T., Çınar, M., Aytemir, M., Tuğlular, I. (1999). Analgesic effect of tianeptine in mice. *Life Sci.* 64: 1313-1319.

Uzbay, I.T., Oglesby, M.W. (2001). Nitric oxide and substance dependence. *Neurosci. Biobehav. Rev.* 25: 43-52.

Uzbay, I.T., Yüksel, N. (2002). Tianeptine in depression treatment. *Journal of Clinical Psychiatry* 5 (Suppl. 2): 10-17 (In Turkish).

Uzbay, I.T. (2004). *Basics of Psychopharmacology and Experimental Technics.* Çizgi Tıp Publishinghouse, Ankara, (In Turkish).

Uzbay, I.T., Çelik, T., Aydın, A., Kayir, H., Tokgöz, S., Bilgi, C. (2004) Effects of chronic ethanol administration and ethanol withdrawal on cyclic guanosine 3',5'-monophosphate (cGMP) levels in the rat brain. *Drug Alcohol. Depend* 74: 55-59.

Uzbay, T. (2005). *Neuroplasticity and Depression.* Çizgi Tıp Publishinghouse, Ankara, (in Turkish).

Uzbay, I.T. (2008). Tianeptine: Potential influences on neuroplasticity and novel pharmacological effects. *Prog. Neuro-Psychopharmacol. Biol. Psychiat.* 32: 915-924.

Vallejo, M. (1994). Transcriptional control of gene expression by cAMP-response element binding proteins. *J. Neuroendocrinol.* 6: 587-596.

van der Hart, M.G., Czéh, B., de Biurrun, G., Michaelis, T., Watanabe, T., Natt, O., Frahm, J., Fuchs, E. (2002). Substance P receptor antagonist and clomipramine prevent stress-induced alterations in cerebral metabolites, cytogenesis in the dentate gyrus and hippocampal volume. *Mol. Psychiatry* 7: 933-941.

van Prag, H., Schinder, A.F., Christie, B.R., Toni, N., Palmer, T.D., Gage, F.H. (2002). Functional neurogenesis in the adult hippocampus. *Nature* 415: 1030-1034.

van Prag, H.M. (1982a). The significance of biological factors in the diagnosis of depressions: I. Biochemical variables. *Comp. Psychiatry* 23: 124-135.

van Prag, H.M. (1982b). Depression, suicide and metabolism of serotonin in the brain. *J. Affect. Dis*. 4: 275-290.

Vaswani, M., Linda, F.K., Ramesh, S. (2003). Role of serotonin reuptake inhibitors in psychiatric disorders: a comprehensive review. *Prog. Neuro-Psychopharmacol. Biol. Psychiat*. 27: 85-102.

Venero, C., Borrel, J. (1999). Rapid glucocorticoid effects on excitatory amino acid levels in the hippocampus: a microdialysis study in freely moving rats. *Eur. J. Neurosci*. 11: 2465-2473.

Vogel, G. (2000). New brain cells prompt new theory of depression. *Science* 290: 258-259.

Vollmann-Honsdorf, G.K., Flügge, G., Fuchs, E. (1997). Chronic psychosocial stress does not affect the number of pyramidal neurons in tree shrew hippocampus. *Neurosci. Lett*. 233: 121-124.

Vouimba, R.M., Munoz, C., Diamond, D.M. (2003). Influence of the antidepressant tianeptine and stress on the expression of synaptic plasticity in the hippocampus and amygdala. *Soc. Neurosci*. 376.6.

Waintraub, L., Septien, L., Azoulay, P. (2000). Efficacy and safety of tianeptine in major depression: evidence from a 3-month controlled clinical trial versus paroxetine. *Eur. Neuropsychopharmacol*, 10 (Suppl. 2): S51.

Watanabe, Y., Gould, E., Daniels, D.C., Cameron, H., McEwen, B.S. (1992). Tianeptine attenuates stress-induced morphological changes in the hippocampus. *Eur. J. Pharmacol*. 222: 157-162.

Wegener, G., Volke, V., Harvey, B.H., Rosenberg, R. (2003). Local, but not systemic, administration of serotonergic antidepressants decreases hippocampal nitric oxide synthase activity. *Brain Res* 959: 128-134.

Wilde, M.I., Benfield, P. (1995). Tianeptine. A review of its pharmacodynamic and pharmacokinetic properties, and therapeutic efficacy in depression and coexisting anxiety and depression. *Drugs* 49: 411-439.

Willner, P. (1985). *Depression. A Psychobiological Synthesis*, New York, Wiley.

Wittenberg, G.M., Tsien, J.Z. (2002) An emerging molecular and cellular framework for memory processing by the hippocampus. *Trends Neurosci.* 25: 501-505.

Woolley, C.S., Gould, E., McEwen, B.S. (1990). Exposure to excess glucocorticoids alters dendritic morphology of adult hippocampal pyramidal neurons. *Brain Res.* 531: 225-231.

Yanik, M., Vural, H., Kocyigit, A., Tutkun, H., Zoroglu, S.S., Herken, H., Savas, H.A., Koylu, A., Akyol, O. (2003) Is the arginine-nitric oxide pathway involved in the pathogenesis of schizophrenia? *Neuropsychobiology* 47: 61-65.

Yaniv, D., Vouimba, R.M., Diamond, D.M., Richter-Levin, G. (2003a). Simultaneous induction of long-term potentiation in the hippocampus and the amygdala by entorhinal cortex activation: mechanistic and temporal profiles. *Neuroscience* 120: 1125-1135.

Yaniv, D., Vouimba, R.M., Diamond, D.M., Richter-Levin, G. (2003b). Effects of novel versus repeated mild stressful experiences on long-term potentiation induced simultaneously in the amygdala and hippocampus in freely behaving rats. *Ann. NY Acad. Sci.* 985: 556-557.

Yin, Q., Kemp, G.J., Yu, L.G., Wagstaff, S.C., Frostick, S.P. (2001a). Expression of Schwann cell-specific proteins and low-molecular-weight neurofilament protein during regeneration of sciatic nerve treated with neurotrophin-4. *Neuroscience* 105: 779-783.

Yin, Q., Kemp, G.J., Yu, L.G., Wagstaff, S.C., Frostick, S.P. (2001b). Neurotrophin-4 delivered by fibrin glue promotes peripheral nerve regeneration. *Muscle Nerve* 24: 345-351.

Yocca, F.D. (1990). Novel Anxiolytic Agents: Actions on Specific Subtypes of Central 5-HT Receptors, *Current and Future Trends in Anticonvulsant, Anxiety and Stroke Therapy*, BS Meldrum, M Williams (Eds.), Wiley-Liss, New York, pp. 145-167.

Zethof, T.J., Van der Heyden, J.A., Tolboom, J.T., Olivier, B. (1995). Stress-induced hyperthermia as a putative anxiety model. Eur J Pharmacol 294: 125-135.

Zoladz, P.R., Park, C.R., Munoz, C., Fleshner, M., Diamond, D.M. (2008). Tianeptine: An antidepressant with memory-protective properties. *Current Neuropharmacology* 6: 311-321.

Zoroglu, S.S., Herken, H., Yurekli, M., Uz, E., Tutkun, H., Savas, H.A., Bagci, C., Ozen, M.E., Cengiz, B., Cakmak, E.A., Dogru, M.I., Akyol, O. (2002). The possible pathophysiological role of plasma nitric oxide and adrenomedullin in schizophrenia. *J. Psychiatr. Res.* 36: 309-315.

Zoroglu, S.S., Yurekli, M., Meram, I., Sogut, S., Tutkun, H., Yetkin, O., Sivasli, E., Savas, H.A., Yanik, M., Herken, H., Akyol, O. (2003). Pathophysiological role of nitric oxide and adrenomedullin in autism. *Cell Biochem. Funct.* 21: 55-60.

Index

N

O

P

T

V

W

Y

U